MEDICAL FINALS:

Structured Answer and Essay Questions

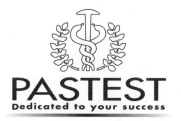

PASTEST
Dedicated to your success

To AJW – an inspirational physician and friend.

Medical Finals:

Structured Answer and Essay Questions

Adam Feather MB MRCP
Lecturer in Clinical Skills,
St. Bartholomew's and the Royal London
School of Medicine and Dentistry
Registrar in Medicine of the Elderly,
Newham General Hospital, London

Ramanathan Visvanathan BM FRCS
Consultant Surgeon, Bronglais General Hospital, Aberystwyth
Honorary Lecturer, University of Wales College of Medicine
Surgical Tutor, Royal College of Surgeons of England
Lately Honorary Senior Lecturer and Assistant Director,
Professorial Surgical Unit, St. Bartholomew's Hospital, London

John S P Lumley MS FRCS
Professor of Surgery, St. Bartholomew's
and the Royal London School of Medicine and Dentistry
Honorary Consultant Surgeon,
St. Bartholomew's Hospital, London
Member of Council, Royal College of Surgeons of England,
Past World President, International College of Surgeons

© 1997 PASTEST
Egerton Court
Parkgate Estate
Knutsford
Cheshire WA16 8DX
Telephone: 01565 752000

First edition 1997
Reprinted 1998, 2000, 2001, 2002, 2003

ISBN: 0 906896 79 7

A catalogue record for this book is available from the British Library.

The information contained within this book was obtained by the authors from reliable sources. However, while every effort has been made to ensure its accuracy, no responsibility for loss, damage or injury occasioned to any person acting or refraining from action as a result of information contained herein can be accepted by the publishers or authors.

Typeset by Breeze Ltd., Manchester.
Printed and bound in Europe by the Alden Group.

CONTENTS

Preface		vi
Revision Checklist		vii
Recommended Reading List		x
How to Use This Book		xi
Abbreviations		xii

SECTION I: Structured Answer Questions

Chapter 1	Infectious Diseases	3
Chapter 2	Metabolic Diseases	15
Chapter 3	Neurology	24
Chapter 4	Endocrinology	40
Chapter 5	Respiratory Medicine	52
Chapter 6	Cardiology	63
Chapter 7	Haematology	74
Chapter 8	Dermatology	82
Chapter 9	Gastroenterology	93
Chapter 10	Nephrology	107
Chapter 11	Rheumatology and Connective Tissue Diseases	117
Chapter 12	Psychiatry	128
Chapter 13	Care of the Elderly	137

SECTION II: SAQ Model Answers and Comments — 145

SECTION III: Essay Writing

Chapter 1	Structured Outlines	295
Chapter 2	Model Essays	302

SECTION IV: Essay Questions — 309

Appendix A: The Medical Finals	318
Appendix B: Self-assessment SAQ Papers	325
Appendix C: Self-assessment Essay Question Papers	326
PasTest Revision Books	327

PREFACE

With the current trend away from traditional essay questions for determining clinical knowledge, more and more examining bodies are introducing structured answer questions (SAQs) into undergraduate and postgraduate medical examinations. SAQs are designed to test problem-solving and decision-making in a structured and objective fashion, and are proving a reliable means of assessing knowledge and understanding in clinical practice. Many examiners also appreciate the fact that SAQs can be marked more quickly, more easily and often more accurately than essays.

This book is intended for undergraduates preparing for their finals and for doctors preparing for the MRCP and MRCGP Part 1 examinations.

Section I consists of SAQs based on medical knowledge in general. The reader is encouraged to write his or her own answers in the boxes provided so that marks can be accurately allocated. Section II contains model answers and marking schedules for every question. The authors have also included short comments to expand on each topic and to highlight common pitfalls that should be avoided. Section III offers advice on how to approach essay questions with a selection of structured outlines to teach good essay planning technique, and several complete genuine sample essays with illuminating examiners' comments. Section IV contains a selection of typical questions to provide invaluable essay writing practice. The three appendices to the book contain additional material likely to be helpful to the reader. Appendix A is an analysis of the final examination in medicine which explains the evolution of assessment techniques and may also be useful to senior doctors who are involved with setting examinations. Appendix B provides the reader with the opportunity to sit mock SAQ examination papers. Each paper provides an authentic mixture of examination topics. Appendix C groups the essay questions in Section IV into mock exam papers.

The book provides a range of questions to be used as a broad base for revision purposes. It may be used as a learning aid, together with medical texts and other information sources, and it is also a valuable method of self-assessment enabling the reader to check his or her progress at each stage of the medical course.

Acknowledgement

We wish to thank Yvonne Mallett for typing the drafts of the text.

REVISION CHECKLIST

Chapter 1: Infection
- ☐ Streptococcal and staphyloccoccal infections
- ☐ Atypical pneumonias
- ☐ Tuberculosis
- ☐ Meningitis
- ☐ Viral hepatitis
- ☐ HIV and associated diseases
- ☐ Sexually transmissable diseases
- ☐ Malaria
- ☐ Parasitic infection

Chapter 2: Metabolic Diseases
- ☐ Wilson's disease
- ☐ Haemochromatosis
- ☐ Porphyria
- ☐ Hyperlipidaemia

Chapter 3: Neurology
- ☐ Strokes – including subarachnoid haemorrhage
- ☐ Epilepsy
- ☐ Multiple sclerosis
- ☐ Parkinson's disease
- ☐ Space occupying lesions
- ☐ Cranial nerve lesions
- ☐ Peripheral neuropathy
- ☐ Cerebellar lesions
- ☐ Myasthenia gravis
- ☐ Motor neurone disease

Chapter 4: Endocrinology
- ☐ Diabetes mellitus
- ☐ Thyrotoxicosis and hypothyroidism
- ☐ Hypothalamic–pituitary–gonadal axis
- ☐ Acromegaly
- ☐ Cushing's syndrome and Addison's disease

Chapter 5: Respiratory Medicine
- ☐ Pneumonia (bacterial and viral)
- ☐ Asthma
- ☐ Pulmonary tuberculosis
- ☐ Chronic bronchitis and emphysema

☐ Bronchogenic carcinoma
☐ Cystic fibrosis and bronchiectasis
☐ Fibrotic lung diseases
☐ Industrial lung diseases

Chapter 6: Cardiology
☐ Ischaemic heart disease
☐ Cardiac failure
☐ Valvular heart disease
☐ Arrhythmias
☐ Endocarditis
☐ Cardiomyopathy

Chapter 7: Haematology
☐ Microcytic and macrocytic anaemia
☐ Haemolytic anaemia
☐ Aplastic anaemia
☐ Leukaemia
☐ Lymphoma
☐ Myeloma
☐ Thrombocytopenia
☐ Bleeding disorders

Chapter 8: Dermatology
☐ Eczema
☐ Psoriasis
☐ Erythema multiforme
☐ Dermatological manifestations of systemic disease
☐ Skin malignancies
☐ Nail disorders
☐ Hair disorders

Chapter 9: Gastroenterology
☐ Dysphagia
☐ Peptic ulcer disease – including *Helicobacter pylori*
☐ Coeliac disease and malabsorptive states
☐ Inflammatory bowel disease
☐ Gastrointestinal bleeds
☐ Viral hepatitis
☐ Alcoholic liver disease
☐ Autoimmune liver disease

Chapter 10: Nephrology
- [ ] Urinary tract infection
- [ ] Nephrotic syndrome
- [ ] Glomerulonephritis
- [ ] Acute and chronic renal failure
- [ ] Diabetic nephropathy
- [ ] Polycystic kidney disease

Chapter 11: Rheumatology and Connective Tissue Disease
- [ ] Rheumatoid arthritis
- [ ] Osteoarthritis
- [ ] Systemic lupus erythematosus
- [ ] Systemic sclerosis
- [ ] Gout and pyrophosphate arthropathy
- [ ] The systemic vasculitides – Wegener's granulomatosis and polyarteritis nodosa
- [ ] Reiter's syndrome
- [ ] Septic arthritis

Chapter 12: Psychiatry
- [ ] Schizophrenia
- [ ] Depression
- [ ] Mania
- [ ] Personality disorder
- [ ] Drug addiction and abuse
- [ ] Alcohol abuse
- [ ] Eating disorders

Chapter 13: Care of the Elderly
- [ ] Falls
- [ ] Dementia and confusional states
- [ ] Incontinence
- [ ] Mobility problems
- [ ] Terminal illness
- [ ] The multidisciplinary team

RECOMMENDED READING LIST

Examining Patients. An Introduction to Clinical Medicine
Toghill PJ, 2nd edition, Edward Arnold, 1995.

Hutchison's Clinical Methods
Hutchison R and Swash M, 21st edition, Saunders, 2001.
This is a guide to clinical medicine combining practical examination methods with background explanation. A classic textbook for all medical students.

Lecture Notes on Clinical Medicine
Rubenstein D, Wayne D and Bradley J, 6th Edition, Blackwell Science, 2002.

Clinical Medicine
Kumar P and Clark M, 5th edition, Saunders, 2002.
This is an excellent undergraduate textbook with useful diagrams, lists and illustrations of the text.

Lecture Notes on Dermatology
Graham-Brown R and Burns T, 8th edition, Blackwell Science, 2002.

Davidson's Principles and Practice of Medicine
Haslett C, Chilvers ER, Boon NA, Colledge NR and Hunter JAA, 19th edition, Churchill Livingstone, 2002.
Has been rather overtaken by *Clinical Medicine* and the *Textbook of Medicine*, but remains a popular and useful guide to clinical medicine.

The Oxford Textbook of Medicine
Warrell DA, Cox TM, Firth JD and Benz Jr EJ, 4th edition, Oxford University Press, 2003.
This book was recently updated and is now presented in three excellent volumes. The layout is much improved and is now easily accessible to undergraduates as well as essential for all postgraduate physicians. It should be used for reference only.

Textbook of Medicine
Souhami RL and Moxham J, 3rd edition, Churchill Livingstone,1997.
Another excellent undergraduate textbook which is comprehensive and well set out.

HOW TO USE THIS BOOK

This book consists of four sections. Sections I and II contain structured answer questions (SAQs) and answers. Sections III and IV contain essay questions and model answers.

Write your answers to the SAQs in the boxes provided. When you have finished, turn to Section II to mark your answers. Allow half marks for incomplete answers, and full marks for sensible and accurate alternatives that the authors have not considered. We hope that the examiners are equally understanding.

Every answer includes a short section of comments which provide concise teaching notes on each topic. Where necessary, refer to the list of recommended textbooks for further information.

At the back of the book, appendices B and C contain typical examination papers enabling you to gain experience of working under timed conditions. Twelve SAQs or four essay questions constitute a two-hour written paper.

Use the Revision Checklist provided to monitor your progress by ticking off subjects with which you feel confident.

ABBREVIATIONS

AAFB   Acid and alcohol fast bacilli
ABGs   Arterial blood gases
ACE   Angiotensin converting enzyme
ACEI   Angiotensin converting enzyme inhibitor
ADLs   Activities of daily living
AF   Atrial fibrillation
AIDS   Acquired immunodeficiency syndrome
ALT   Alanine aminotransferase
ANCA   Antinuclear cytoplasmic antibody (p = perinuclear,
        c = cytoplasmic)
ANF   Antinuclear factor
ASOT   Antistreptolysin O titre
AST   Aspartate transaminase
AXR   Abdominal X-ray

BCG   Bacille Calmette–Guérin
BM   Glucose blood monitoring
BMI   Body mass index

Ca   Carcinoma
CAH   Chronic active hepatitis
CAPD   Continuous ambulatory peritoneal dialysis
CCU   Coronary care unit
CK-MB   Creatine kinase-myocardium and brain isoenzyme
CMV   Cytomegalovirus
CNS   Central nervous system
CPK   Creatine phosphokinase
CSU   Catheter specimen of urine
CVA   Cerebrovascular accident
CXR   Chest X-ray

DC   Direct current
DCCT   Diabetic control and complications trial
DEXA   Dual X-ray absorptiometry
DIC   Disseminated intravascular coagulopathy
DNA   Deoxyribonucleic acid
DSA   Digital subtraction angiography
DVT   Deep vein thrombosis

ECG   Electrocardiogram

E. coli	*Esherichia coli*
EBV	Epstein–Barr virus
EEG	Electroencephalogram
EMG	Electromyelogram
ESR	Erythrocyte sedimentation rate
FBC	Full blood count
FDPs	Fibrinogen degradation products
Fe	Iron
FEV	Forced expiratory volume
Fl	Femtolitres
FFP	Fresh frozen plasma
FSH	Follicle stimulating hormone
FVC	Forced vital capacity
GABA	Gamma aminobutyric acid
GCS	Glasgow coma scale
GI	Gastrointestinal
GIT	Gastrointestinal tract
GP	General practitioner
GTN	Glyceryl trinitrate
GUSTO	Global utilization of streptokinase and tPA for occlusive coronary artery disease trial
HB/Hb	Haemoglobin
HBV	Hepatitis B virus
HCV	Hepatitis C virus
HIV	Human immunodeficiency virus
HLA	Human leucocyte antigen
HRT	Hormone replacement therapy
HSV	Herpes simplex virus
HUS	Haemolytic uraemic syndrome
ICD	International classification of disease
IDDM	Insulin dependent diabetes mellitus
IDL	Intermediate density lipoprotein
Ig	Immunoglobulin
IHD	Ischaemic heart disease
IM	Intramuscular
IQ	Intelligence quotient
ITU	Intensive care unit

IV	Intravenous
IVU	Intravenous urography
Kg	Kilogrammes
LDL	Low density lipoprotein
LFTs	Liver function tests
LMN	Lower motor neurone lesion
LH	Luteinising hormone
MAOI	Monoamine oxidase inhibitor
MCH	Mean corpuscular haemoglobin
MCHC	Mean corpuscular haemoglobin concentration
MC+S	Microscopy, culture and sensitivity
MCV	Mean corpuscular volume
MDRTB	Multidrug resistant tuberculosis
MI	Myocardial infarction
MRI	Magnetic resonance imaging
MST	Morphine sulphate tablets
MSU	Midstream urine
NSAIDs	Non-steroidal anti-inflammatory drugs
NSU	Non-specific urethritis
OGD	Oesophagogastroduodenoscopy
PAN	Polyarteritis nodosa
PCWP	Pulmonary capillary wedge pressure
PEFR	Peak expiratory flow rate
PNS	Peripheral nervous system
PRV	Polycythaemia rubra vera
PVD	Peripheral vascular disease
SIADH	Syndrome of inappropiate antidiuretic hormone
SLE	Systemic lupus erythrematosus
Spp	Species
STD	Sexually transmissable disease
SVT	Supraventricular tachycardia
TB	Tuberculosis
TENS	Transcutaneous electrical nerve stimulation

TIA	Transient ischaemic attack
TIBC	Total iron binding capacity
TFTs	Thyroid function tests
tPA	Tissue plasminogen activator
TURP	Transurethral resection of the prostate
U&Es	Urea and electrolytes
UK	United Kingdom
UKPDS	United Kingdom Prospective Diabetic Study
UMN	Upper motor neurone lesion
USS	Ultrasound scan
UTI	Urinary tract infection
VLDL	Very low density lipoprotein
VF	Ventricular fibrillation
VQ	VQ ventilation/perfusion scan
VT	Ventricular tachycardia
WHO	World Health Organization
WW	World War

SECTION I:
STRUCTURED ANSWER QUESTIONS

CHAPTER 1: INFECTIOUS DISEASES

Question 1

A 29-year-old Thai restaurateur presents to his GP with a three-month history of worsening jaundice and right upper quadrant pain. As an infant in Thailand he had been jaundiced, but had enjoyed good health until this present episode.

(a) What is the likely cause of his jaundice? (1 mark)

(b) List three modes of acquiring this disorder. (3 marks)

(c) Briefly outline your investigations and therapeutic management. (6 marks)

Question 2

A 13-year-old schoolgirl presents to the Accident and Emergency department with a five-day history of an upper respiratory tract infection, now complicated by a severe headache, photophobia and neck stiffness. Her mother has also noticed a rapidly developing purpuric rash over her legs in the last few hours.

(a)   State the diagnosis, and list two possible causative organisms. (3 marks)

(b)   List six investigations you would perform. (3 marks)

(c)   Briefly outline your therapeutic management. (4 marks)

Question 3

A 46-year-old woman returns from Bangladesh after a three-month visit to see her family. Whilst in Bangladesh she developed night sweats, a productive cough, with green sputum and occasional haemoptysis. In the last two weeks she has also developed diarrhoea and has lost several kilogrammes in weight.

(a) What is the likely organism causing her symptoms? (1 mark)

(b) List five investigations you would perform in this case to confirm the diagnosis. (5 marks)

(c) List the drugs which may be used in this case, with a side effect of each. (4 marks)

Question 4

A 36-year-old man presents to his GP three days after returning from a business trip to Nigeria, with a five-day history of fever, malaise and rigors. He denies any other systemic upset and has not taken any antimalarial prophylaxis.

(a)   List three species of malaria and three drugs used in the treatment. (3 marks)

(b)   List three investigations you would perform. (3 marks)

(c)   Outline the advice you would have given this man if he had come to see you prior to his trip. (4 marks)

Question 5

A 17-year-old schoolgirl presents to her GP with a two-week history of worsening pharyngitis associated with flu-like symptoms and swelling of the lymph nodes in her neck. On examination she has a petechial rash over her soft palate, tender cervical lymphadenopathy, and splenomegaly, with the spleen palpable 2 cm below the left costal margin.

(a)   State the most likely infectious cause of her symptoms and give two alternative diagnoses. (3 marks)

(b)   List five investigations you would perform. (5 marks)

(c)   Outline your management. (2 marks)

Question 6

A 27-year-old man with a previously known AIDS-defining illness, presents to the Accident and Emergency department with a 48-hour history of worsening confusion, headache and right-sided limb weakness.

(a)   List three AIDS-defining illnesses. (3 marks)

(b)   Give two possible causes of his symptoms. (2 marks)

(c)   Outline the investigations you would perform. (5 marks)

Question 7

A 24-year-old businessman returns from Bangkok with a one-week history of a painful urethral discharge, and a painless ulcerative lesion on the glans of his penis.

(a)   (i)   What is the term used to describe the lesion on his penis? (1 mark)

        (ii)   List two organisms that may be responsible for his symptoms. (2 marks)

(b)   Give three other examples of infectious diseases that may be acquired in a similar manner. (3 marks)

(c)   Outline your investigations and therapeutic management. (4 marks)

Question 8

A 21-year-old man presents to the Accident and Emergency department with an eight-hour history of diarrhoea and abdominal cramps, after eating some poorly thawed chicken at a barbecue.

(a)   (i)   What is the condition he is suffering from? (1 mark)

       (ii)   List three organisms that could be responsible. (3 marks)

(b)   Give two other risk factors for contracting such an illness. (2 marks)

(c)   Briefly outline your investigations and therapeutic management. (4 marks)

Question 9

A 59-year-old man is recovering five days after an elective right total hip replacement. He has an indwelling urinary catheter *in situ* and an intravenous cannula in each forearm. During the last 24 hours he has become increasingly unwell, with a swinging pyrexia. He is now clammy and pale, with a pulse of 110 and a blood pressure of 80/60.

(a) (i) What is the term used to describe his condition? (1 mark)
     (ii) List three possible causes in this man's case. (3 marks)

(b) List six essential investigations you would perform. (3 marks)

(c) Briefly outline your management. (3 marks)

Question 10

A 21-year-old female nurse returns from working in India with a two-month history of diarrhoea, now associated with episodic rigors and right upper quadrant pain. She also complains of an irritating pain in her right shoulder. Stool culture and microscopy reveal cysts.

(a)   What is the diagnosis and the causative organism? (2 marks)

(b)   What is the cause of her right upper quadrant pain? How is it related to her shoulder pain? (2 marks)

(c)   (i)   List three investigations you would perform in this case. (3 marks)

        (ii)   Outline the therapeutic options. (3 marks)

Question 11

A 27-year-old man returns after a two-year period working in Thailand, with a three-month history of intermittent abdominal pain, diarrhoea and a dry cough associated with wheezing. During this period he has lost 5 kg in weight. A full blood count organised by his GP shows a normal white cell count but with a 'gross eosinophilia'.

(a)   (i)   What is the likely group of organisms responsible for his eosinophilia? (1 mark)

        (ii)   List two other causes of an eosinophilia. (2 marks)

(b)   What is the cause of his respiratory symptoms? (2 marks)

(c)   Briefly outline your investigations and therapeutic management. (5 marks)

Question 12

A 19-year-old student returns from a caving holiday in the southern states of America with a two-week history of fever, a non-productive cough and arthralgia. His GP sends him to the chest clinic where a diagnosis of histoplasmosis is made.

(a)　(i)　　What type of organism is Histoplasma? (1 mark)
　　　(ii)　　List two more common conditions that are caused by this group of organisms. (2 marks)

(b)　List three investigations you would perform. (3 marks)

(c)　List four drugs used in the treatment of such infections, with a side effect of each. (4 marks)

CHAPTER 2: METABOLIC DISEASES

Question 1

A 16-year-old schoolboy presents to the medical outpatient department with a three-month history of neurological symptoms, including tremor, and choreiform movements, associated with behavioural problems at school. On examination he has several stigmata of chronic liver disease, and greyish rings are noted around the cornea. A clinical diagnosis of Wilson's disease is made.

(a)   What is the name given to the grey corneal rings and which trace element is associated with this disorder? (2 marks)

(b)   List three investigations that would confirm the clinical diagnosis. (3 marks)

(c)   Outline your therapeutic management. (5 marks)

Question 2

A 36-year-old man presents to his GP with a three-month history of polyuria and polydypsia, associated with painful swelling of both knees. On examination he has a suntanned appearance (despite not having been in the sun for several months), and has several signs of chronic liver disease, with 5 cm hepatomegaly below the right costal margin. He also has arthritis of both knees.

(a)   State the diagnosis and the causative factor. (3 marks)

(b)   List five investigations you would perform. (4 marks)

(c)   What is the cause of:-
        (i)   the polyuria and polydypsia?
        (ii)   his suntanned appearance?
        (iii)   the arthritis? (3 marks)

Question 3

A 27-year-old man is found to have a cholesterol of 11.0 mmol/l with normal triglycerides, at a routine insurance medical examination. On direct questioning he says that his father and uncle, both non-smokers, died in their early 40s of ischaemic heart disease.

(a) Which inherited disorder does this man have and what is its mode of inheritance? (2 marks)

(b) List two clinical signs you would look for in association with this cholesterol level, and two bedside tests you would perform. (4 marks)

(c) Briefly outline your management. (4 marks)

Question 4

A 2-year-old boy with known glucose-6-phosphatase deficiency presents in the paediatric outpatient department with increasing lethargy and general ill health. On examination he is of short stature and obese; he has hepatomegaly and palpable kidneys.

(a)   Of which group of disorders is this disease an example? (2 marks)

(b)   What is its mode of inheritance? Give three other examples. (4 marks)

(c)   If this patient was presenting for the first time, how would you attempt to confirm the diagnosis (definitive tests are not required). (4 marks)

Chapter 2: Metabolic Diseases

Question 5

A 20-year-old woman presents to the Accident and Emergency department with a six-hour history of acute abdominal pain. She denies any gastrointestinal or urogenital symptoms, but says she has had two less severe, similar episodes in the last few months since starting the oral contraceptive pill. The medical registrar makes a clinical diagnosis of acute porphyria.

(a) Give two further symptoms that may be presenting features. (2 marks)

(b) List three other precipitating factors. (3 marks)

(c) Outline your therapeutic management. (5 marks)

Question 6

A 3-year-old boy is brought to the paediatric outpatient department by his parents, who are both Ashkenazi Jews. The boy has been unwell for several months complaining of left upper quadrant pain. On examination he is clinically anaemic, has a greyish pigmentation and has multiple bruises over his back and forearms. He is also noted to have hepatomegaly and massive splenomegaly. A clinical diagnosis of Gaucher's disease is made.

(a)   List two other disorders that are common amongst Ashkenazi Jews. (2 marks)

(b)   (i)   To which group of disorders does Gaucher's disease belong and what is its mode of inheritance? (2 marks)

        (ii)   List three investigations that are indicated from the history. (3 marks)

(c)   Outline your advice to the parents with regard to treatment and prognosis. (3 marks)

Question 7

A 21-year-old man with known homocystinuria presents to the Accident and Emergency department with a 36-hour history of increasing pain and swelling in the left calf, now associated with shortness of breath and an episode of haemoptysis. On examination he has Marfanoid features with pectus carinatum.

(a)   What is the mode of inheritance of this disorder? (1 mark)

(b)   List three Marfanoid features and explain the term pectus carinatum. (4 marks)

(c)   What is the presenting complication in this case? Briefly outline your therapeutic management. (5 marks)

Question 8

A previously healthy 17-year-old girl was admitted to the Accident and Emergency department following an overdose of aspirin. On examination she was semi-conscious, hypotensive and oliguric.

(a)   List the metabolic effects of salicylate toxicity. (3 marks)

(b)   How would you correct the metabolic deficit? (4 marks)

(c)   List three other drugs with similar toxic effects. (3 marks)

Question 9

A 29-year-old female athlete collapsed during the London Marathon. She was taken to Accident and Emergency where she was found to be conscious but hyperventilating and hypotensive.

(a)   State the main physiological events that had overcome the patient and their underlying mechanisms. (4 marks)

(b)   List the immediate resuscitatory measures required. (2 marks)

(c)   How would you assess and correct the underlying metabolic disorder? (4 marks)

CHAPTER 3: NEUROLOGY

Question 1

A 74-year-old man is sent to the Accident and Emergency department by his GP with a 6–7 hour history of weakness affecting his left upper and lower limbs, and the left side of his face. He also complains of slurring of his speech.

(a) What is the diagnosis, and which blood vessel is most likely to be involved? (2 marks)

(b) List the clinical features you would use to differentiate an upper and a lower motor neurone weakness. (2 marks)

(c) List the essential investigations you would perform (3 marks) and outline your further management. (3 marks)

Chapter 3: Neurology

Question 2

A 19-year-old secretary presents to the Accident and Emergency department with a six-hour history of a severe headache. The headache came on suddenly whilst she was at work. She says she feels as though "someone has hit me over the back of the head with a baseball bat". She has been nauseated with mild neck stiffness, but denies fever or photophobia.

(a)   What is the likely cause of her headache? (1 mark)

(b)   Give three other causes of a severe headache in this case. (3 marks)

(c)   Briefly outline your investigations and therapeutic management. (6 marks)

Question 3

A 59-year-old smoker presents to his GP with a four-month history of a cough, episodic haemoptysis, and a 10 kg weight loss. On examination he has a partial ptosis of the right eye associated with enophthalmos and a constricted pupil. Respiratory examination reveals coarse crackles and bronchial breathing in the right upper zone.

(a)   What is the eponymous syndrome associated with this man's eye signs, and what is the neurological lesion involved? (2 marks)

(b)   (i)   What is the probable cause of the syndrome in this case? (1 mark)

        (ii)   List three other causes. (3 marks)

(c)   Another patient presents with a full ptosis and fixed dilated pupil of the right eye. The eye is facing down and out. Explain neurologically the appearances of the eye and list two causes. (4 marks)

Question 4

A 47-year-old woman presents to her GP with a two-day history of a weakness affecting the left side of her face. She has no other neurological deficit and is otherwise well.

(a)   (i)   Which cranial nerve has been affected? (1 mark)

        (ii)   How would you differentiate between an upper and a lower motor neurone lesion? (2 marks)

(b)   List four causes of this cranial nerve palsy. (4 marks)

(c)   It is suspected this is an idiopathic lower motor neurone lesion. What is the eponymous name of this lesion? Briefly outline your management. (3 marks)

Question 5

A 36-year-old man with known poorly controlled insulin dependent diabetes mellitus, presents in the diabetic clinic with a three-month history of worsening numbness and parasthesiae in his hands and feet, associated with a large ulcer on the sole of his left heel.

(a) (i)   What is the probable cause of his symptoms? (1 mark)
     (ii) List two other causes. (2 marks)

(b) List the modalities of sensation you would test and the spinal tracts in which they are carried. (3 marks)

(c) List four other neurological complications of diabetes mellitus. (4 marks)

Question 6

A 26-year-old woman presents to her GP with a two-month history of early morning headaches. The headaches are constant, but far worse in the mornings and when she laughs or coughs. Initially they were relieved by aspirin but now nothing seems to make the headache better. More recently she has been nauseated and has had some blurring of her vision.

(a)   List three possible causes of her headache. (3 marks)

(b)   Give three essential investigations you would perform in this case. (3 marks)

(c)   Outline the therapeutic options. (4 marks)

Question 7

A 20-year-old female student presents in the neurology outpatient department with a three-month history of 'funny turns' lasting 2–3 minutes. Each is preceded by an 'odd sensation', and is followed by a feeling of 'vacancy'. She has no recollection of these events, but has been told about them by her friends, who say she becomes vacant and unresponsive, with grinding of her teeth and contortion of her face.

(a)   What is the likely cause of her 'turns'? (1 mark)

(b)   List five investigations you would perform. (5 marks)

(c)   List four therapeutic agents that may be used in this case, giving a side effect of each. (4 marks)

Question 8

A 57-year-old man is seen in the neurology outpatients department with a four-month history of wasting of his upper and lower limbs, associated with progressive worsening of his mobility. More recently he has also had 'difficulty' with his speech and 'choking' whilst eating and drinking.

(a) What is the underlying diagnosis, and the reason for his 'difficulty' with speech and 'choking' when eating? (3 marks)

(b) List three investigations relevant to this case. (3 marks)

(c) List the management strategies you would use. (4 marks)

Question 9

A 29-year-old woman presents to her GP with a four-month history of shoulder and hip weakness, particularly with exercise. She has also noticed blurring of her vision and difficulty with chewing, particularly towards the end of a long meal. The most striking feature on examination is marked bilateral ptosis, with weakness of the extra-ocular muscles.

(a)   State the diagnosis and its pathogenesis. (3 marks)

(b)   List two investigations you would perform. (2 marks)

(c)   List the therapeutic options you would employ. (5 marks)

Question 10

A 62-year-old man presents to the medical outpatients department with a one-year history of progressive difficulty in walking and falls. He has developed a marked tremor of both hands and has noticed that his writing is becoming increasingly 'shaky and small'.

(a) What is the diagnosis and the neurotransmitter involved in this condition? (2 marks)

(b) List two other conditions that may present in a similar manner. (2 marks)

(c) List three drugs that may be used in this case and a recognized side effect of each. (6 marks)

Question 11

A 3-year-old boy presents in the paediatric clinic with repeated falls, poor walking and an inability to climb on to furniture or up the stairs. A clinical diagnosis of Duchenne's muscular dystrophy is made.

(a)　(i)　How is this disorder classically inherited? (1 mark)

　　　(ii)　List two other examples of this type of inheritance. (2 marks)

(b)　List three investigations to confirm the clinical diagnosis in this patient. (3 marks)

(c)　List four other causes of proximal muscle weakness. (4 marks)

Question 12

A 26-year-old man is sent to the neurology outpatient department by his GP with an eight-week history of numbness and parasthesiae in his hands and feet, associated with an episode of blurred vision and pain in the left eye which resolved spontaneously.

(a) What is the underlying diagnosis, and what is the pathological basis of the disorder? (2 marks)

(b) List three investigations you would perform and the expected abnormalities. (3 marks)

(c) Briefly outline your management once the diagnosis is confirmed. (5 marks)

Question 13

A 62-year-old woman presents to the Accident and Emergency department with a two-week history of increasing weakness and numbness in her lower limbs, associated with difficulty in passing urine and constipation. She had a Dukes C carcinoma of the colon treated 18 months previously. On examination she has a spastic paraparesis and a sensory loss at level T10.

(a)   (i)   What is the likely cause of the spastic paraparesis in this case? (1 mark)

      (ii)   List two other causes. (2 marks)

(b)   Define the surface anatomy of a T10 sensory level and list three essential investigations you would perform to confirm the lesion and its level. (4 marks)

(c)   Outline your management strategy. (3 marks)

Question 14

A 27-year-old man presents to the Accident and Emergency department with a 10-day history of an upper respiratory tract infection, now associated with increasing weakness and numbness in the lower limbs. On examination he has lower motor neurone signs in his lower limbs associated with sensory loss to the level of the upper thighs.

(a)   (i)   What is the cause of this man's sensorimotor neuropathy? (1 mark)

       (ii)   List two other causes. (2 marks)

(b)   List the lower motor neurone signs you would elicit. (3 marks)

(c)   Outline your therapeutic management. (4 marks)

Question 15

A 45-year-old man is brought to the neurology outpatient department by his wife, with an eight-month history of increasing forgetfulness, inappropriately aggressive behaviour and a generalized change in his personality. More recently he has had 'writhing' and 'lunging' movements of the arms and legs. His wife thinks his father also had a similar problem. A clinical diagnosis of Huntington's chorea is made.

(a)   How is this disorder inherited and what are the chances of this man's offspring being affected? (2 marks)

(b)   Define what is meant by chorea, and give two other causes. (4 marks)

(c)   Briefly outline your management. (4 marks)

Question 16

A 49-year-old man, who is a known chronic alcohol abuser, presents to the Accident and Emergency department with a two-day history of worsening tremor and decreased mobility. He has been on phenytoin for 2 years after sustaining a head injury whilst inebriated. On examination he has several stigmata of chronic liver disease and gross cerebellar signs. He is not encephalopathic.

(a)   List four cerebellar signs you may expect to elicit. (2 marks)

(b)   Give two causes of the cerebellar syndrome in this patient. (2 marks)

(c)   List three investigations you would perform and three drugs you would prescribe in this man's further management. (6 marks)

CHAPTER 4: ENDOCRINOLOGY

Question 1

A 67-year-old woman gives a history of listlessness, inactivity and weight gain over several months. Her serum thyroxine level is low, and thyroid stimulating hormone raised (> 20 mU/l).

(a) (i)   State the clinical diagnosis. (1 mark)
     (ii) List four causes of this condition. (2 marks)

(b) Discuss the therapeutic management of this patient. (3 marks)

(c) Before treatment could commence, the patient was found unconscious at home. Discuss your management. (4 marks)

Question 2

A 31-year-old woman is referred to the medical clinic with a history of heat intolerance, fatigue and palpitations. On examination she has a fine finger tremor and bulging eyes.

(a) State the probable clinical diagnosis and its pathogenesis. (3 marks)

(b) List the other clinical findings that would confirm your diagnosis. (3 marks)

(c) List the treatment modalities available and their complications. (4 marks)

Question 3

A 36-year-old woman is referred to the endocrinology clinic with a history of headaches, oligomenorrhoea and infertility. Her serum prolactin levels are persistently elevated; she is not on any medication.

(a)   (i)   State the diagnosis. (1 mark)

        (ii)   List two physiological states where plasma prolactin levels are raised. (2 marks)

(b)   List four drugs that may elevate plasma prolactin. (3 marks)

(c)   How would you treat this condition? (4 marks)

Question 4

A 40-year-old woman is referred to the endocrine clinic with a four-month history of tunnel vision, joint pains and slurring of speech. She recently had to change her shoes and gloves for larger sizes.

(a)   (i)   State the clinical diagnosis and the pathology of the lesion. (2 marks)

       (ii)   How would you confirm the diagnosis biochemically? (2 marks)

(b)   List other clinical features that characterize this disease. (3 marks)

(c)   List the methods of treating this condition. (3 marks)

Question 5

A 35-year-old woman with muscle weakness, skin bruising, hypertension and an impaired glucose tolerance is diagnosed as having Cushing's syndrome.

(a)   What is the cause of this syndrome? (2 marks)

(b)   State the basis of the four findings stated. (4 marks)

(c)   State the biochemical investigations needed to establish the cause of this syndrome. (4 marks)

Question 6

A 58-year-old woman with a history of weight loss, malaise, weakness and increased skin pigmentation is found to be suffering from adrenal cortical insufficiency.

(a)   State the causes of this condition. (3 marks)

(b)   List the other clinical features associated with this condition. (3 marks)

(c)   Name two biochemical tests required to confirm the clinical diagnosis. (4 marks)

Question 7

A 60-year-old Afro-Caribbean male presents with muscle weakness, poly-uria and polydipsia. A diagnosis of primary hyperaldosteronism is made.

(a)   State the pathophysiology of this disease. (3 marks)

(b)   State two biochemical findings. (2 marks)

(c)   State the principles of treatment. (3 marks)

(d)   What is meant by secondary hyperaldosteronism? (2 marks)

Question 8

(a)   How does anti-diuretic hormone (vasopressin) regulate the sensation of thirst? (3 marks)

(b)   What is diabetes insipidus and how does it present? (3 marks)

(c)   Discuss the treatment of this disease. (4 marks)

Question 9

A 70-year-old woman is admitted as an emergency with nausea, vomiting, polyuria and drowsiness. Her serum calcium level is 4.2 mmol/l.

(a)   What is she suffering from that requires urgent treatment? (2 marks)

(b)   List six disease states not involving the parathyroid glands that are associated with this condition. (3 marks)

(c)   Discuss the immediate measures required to lower her serum calcium level. (5 marks)

Question 10

A 49-year-old man complains of paroxysmal attacks of headache, palpitations, vomiting, breathlessness and weakness, and says he felt he was 'going to die' during the episodes. Clinically he is pale and hypertensive.

(a)   List four differential diagnoses that would fit the above findings. (2 marks)

(b)   His plasma catecholamine assay is > 1000 μg/ml.
  (i)   State the diagnosis. (2 marks)
  (ii)   How would you localize the lesion? (3 marks)

(c)   Outline your treatment. (3 marks)

Question 11

A 24-year-old woman presents to her GP with a four-month history of polydypsia, polyuria, recurrent vaginal candidiasis and weight loss. A BM measurement is 17–28.

(a)   What is the diagnosis? (2 marks)

(b)   How would you confirm the diagnosis? (4 marks)

(c)   Outline patient education in managing her disease. (4 marks)

Question 12

A 58-year-old poorly controlled non-insulin dependent diabetic man is brought to the Accident and Emergency department in a comatosed state.

(a)   Give four causes of diabetic coma. (2 marks)

(b)   List six complications of poorly controlled diabetes. (3 marks)

(c)   Outline your investigation and treatment of hyperglycaemic coma. (5 marks)

CHAPTER 5: RESPIRATORY MEDICINE

Question 1

A 17-year-old male student with known asthma attends the Accident and Emergency department with a three-day history of a cough productive of yellow sputum, worsening shortness of breath and wheeze.

(a)   Give two reaons why a chest X-ray must be performed. (2 marks)

(b)   List three other investigations you would perform. (3 marks)

(c)   (i)   List the criteria you would use to assess the severity of this asthma exacerbation. (2 marks)

         (ii)   Briefly outline your initial therapeutic management. (3 marks)

Question 2

A 26-year-old woman presents to her GP with a three-day history of a dry cough and exertional dyspnoea. A chest X-ray is arranged and reveals 'patchy consolidation' in the right upper lobe for which she is started on amoxycillin. Over the next 48 hours she continues to deteriorate and is subsequently admitted to hospital.

(a)   What is the descriptive term given to this woman's condition? (1 mark)

(b)   List four causative organisms that may be implicated. (4 marks)

(c)   State an expected abnormality in each of the following investigations:
(i) FBC (ii) U+Es (iii) LFTs (iv) ABGs (v) Immune markers. (5 marks)

Question 3

A 63-year-old man who is a lifelong smoker, attends the chest clinic with a 2–3 year history of worsening exertional dyspnoea, associated with a productive cough. He is prone to chest infections during the winter months.

(a) Outline the important points you would need to elucidate in the history. (5 marks)

(b) List three non-haematological investigations you would do in this case. (3 marks)

(c) List four drugs that may be employed in this case. (2 marks)

Question 4

A 61-year-old man presents to his GP with a four-month history of a cough associated with episodic fresh haemoptysis. During this period he has lost 5 kg in weight despite a reasonable appetite. He is a lifelong smoker.

(a)   What is the most likely diagnosis? (1 mark)

(b)   List three investigations to confirm the diagnosis. (3 marks)

(c)   Describe the various treatment options. (6 marks)

Question 5

A 28-year-old woman presents to the Accident and Emergency department with a six-hour history of sudden onset of severe, right-sided pleuritic chest pain, associated with shortness of breath and an episode of haemoptysis.

(a)   What is the most likely diagnosis? (1 mark)

(b)   List six risk factors for this disease. (3 marks)

(c)   (i)   Outline the investigations you would perform. (3 marks)
         (ii)   Briefly outline the therapeutic management. (3 marks)

Question 6

A 30-year-old Afro-Caribbean woman presents to her GP with a six-month history of exertional dyspnoea, and a painful red lesion on her shin. She also complains of dry itchy eyes. A clinical diagnosis of sarcoidosis is made.

(a)   What is the painful red lesion on her shin, and what is the term used to describe her eye condition? (2 marks)

(b)   List three other extra-pulmonary manifestations of sarcoidosis. (3 marks)

(c)   List the essential investigations to confirm the diagnosis. (5 marks)

Question 7

A 16-year-old schoolboy with a known chronic chest condition presents to his GP with a three-month history of worsening malaise, lethargy and loose, offensive, porridge-like stools. On examination he is pale and cachectic, with marked clubbing of his fingernails. Respiratory examination reveals an expiratory wheeze associated with coarse bibasal crackles and production of copious amounts of green sputum. His BM is 17–28.

(a) What is the chronic underlying disorder? (1 mark)

(b) Which three complications have developed? (3 marks)

(c) List the long term management strategies you would employ in the management. (6 marks)

Question 8

A 55-year-old man presents to the chest clinic with a 12-month history of worsening exertional dyspnoea associated with an irritating dry cough. On examination he has clubbing of the fingernails and fine inspiratory crepitations are heard in the lower zones of both lung fields.

(a)   What is the diagnosis? (1 mark)

(b)   List three disorders that may present or are associated with this diagnosis. (3 marks)

(c)   List three investigations to confirm the diagnosis and the expected abnormality with each. (6 marks)

Question 9

A 66-year-old retired boiler lagger presents to his GP with a three-month history of worsening shortness of breath and, more recently, a cough with episodic haemoptysis. He is a lifelong smoker.

(a) To which group of pulmonary disorders does this man's underlying condition belong? Give two other examples. (3 marks)

(b) What is the most likely cause of his shortness of breath and the haemoptysis? (2 marks)

(c) List the radiological features that may be seen on this man's chest X-ray. (5 marks)

Question 10

A 32-year-old farm labourer presents to his GP with a six-month history of episodic shortness of breath associated with a flu-like illness. His symptoms are particularly prevalent when he is working with hay and straw.

(a)   What is the condition from which he is suffering and to which group of pulmonary disorders does it belong? (2 marks)

(b)   List four agents or sources that have been implicated in the causation of these disorders. (4 marks)

(c)   Briefly outline your advice to this man if he decides to continue farming. (4 marks)

Question 11

A 21-year-old female student is hit by a car whilst cycling home from college. She sustains multiple fractures which are surgically reduced. During the post-operative 48 hours, her respiratory function worsens insidiously, and after review by the medical registrar she is electively intubated and ventilated.

(a)   What is the term used to describe her respiratory problem? (1 mark)

(b)   Give two diagnostic criteria. (2 marks)

(c)   (i)   List six essential investigations you would perform. (3 marks)
       (ii)   Briefly outline your management prior to her being ventilated. (4 marks)

CHAPTER 6: CARDIOLOGY

Question 1

A 47-year-old man presents to Accident and Emergency department with a four-hour history of severe central chest pain radiating to his neck and arms. He is sweaty, nauseated and has felt dizzy and faint.

(a)   (i)   What is the most likely diagnosis? (1 mark)

        (ii)   List six major risk factors. (2 marks)

(b)   List three drugs which have been proven to improve prognosis in this condition. (3 marks)

(c)   Briefly outline your management. (4 marks)

Question 2

Six weeks after an acute anterior myocardial infarction, a 47-year-old man is seen in the medical outpatients department. Since discharge he has remained asymptomatic. Investigations whilst he was an inpatient show: glucose 15.4 mmol/l, cholesterol 7.6 mmol/l, normal triglycerides, echocardiogram 'moderately impaired left ventricular function'.

(a)   List four drugs you would ensure this man was taking. (4 marks)

(b)   Which other department in the hospital must he attend? (1 mark)

(c)   Briefly outline your further management. (5 marks)

Question 3

A 64-year-old retired headmistress presents to her GP with a three-month history of exertional dyspnoea, swelling of her ankles and orthopnoea even with three pillows at night. In the past she has had two myocardial infarctions, and remains on treatment for longstanding hypertension.

(a)   Name two medications she may be taking which could be exacerbating her symptoms. (2 marks)

(b)   List the radiological features that may be evident on a CXR. (4 marks)

(c)   Briefly outline your management for this woman. (4 marks)

Question 4

A 71-year-old retired policeman attends the medical outpatient department with a three-month history of episodic fast, irregular palpitations, associated with shortness of breath. On one occasion his left upper and lower limbs became weak, but this resolved spontaneously. He smokes 10 cigarettes per day and drinks a half bottle of whisky every two days.

(a) (i)   What is the likely tachyarrhythmia causing his symptoms? (1 mark)

(ii) List two conditions that may be responsible for his arrythmia, and his risk factors for developing them. (2 marks)

(b) What is the term used to describe the limb weakness? (2 marks)

(c) Outline your management in this case. (5 marks)

Question 5

A 48-year-old factory manager presents to the Accident and Emergency department with a three-week history of exertional dyspnoea, malaise and fever. During the 48 hours prior to presentation he has been in bed with a flu-like illness and a dry cough. His wife comments that his ankles have swelled markedly during this period. On examination he has a harsh pansystolic murmur, principally in the mitral area.

(a)   (i)   What is the underlying diagnosis? (1 mark)

        (ii)   List three eponymous signs associated with the diagnosis, explaining what they are. (3 marks)

(b)   Give two essential investigations you would perform. (2 marks)

(c)   List the complications that may occur. (4 marks)

Question 6

A 36-year-old keen amateur sportsman presents to the cardiology clinic with a six-month history of exertional dyspnoea, and chest pains, associated with one episode of collapse whilst out jogging. Of note his father had 'dropped dead' whilst playing football.

(a) What is the underlying cardiac condition and how is it inherited? (2 marks)

(b) List three other causes of cardiomyopathy. (3 marks)

(c) Briefly outline your investigations and management. (5 marks)

Question 7

A 16-year-old schoolgirl presents to outpatients with worsening exertional dyspnoea. On examination she has marked clubbing of her fingernails and is cyanosed at rest. Cardiovascular examination reveals a parasternal heave and an ejection systolic murmur, heard predominantly in the pulmonary area.

(a)   Give three causes of cyanotic heart disease. (3 marks)

(b)   What are the four components of Fallot's tetralogy? (4 marks)

(c)   Briefly outline the treatment options. (3 marks)

Question 8

A 59-year-old woman becomes acutely short of breath two days after an acute myocardial infarction.

(a)   List three possible causes for her shortness of breath. (3 marks)

(b)   Give six investigations you would perform immediately. (3 marks)

(c)   Briefly outline your management of the most likely diagnosis. (4 marks)

Question 9

A 64-year-old man presents in the cardiology clinic with a two-year history of exertional chest pain and associated dyspnoea. More recently he has had three syncopal episodes whilst out walking his dog.

(a)   (i)   What is the cardiac valvular lesion causing his symptoms? (1 mark)

       (ii)   List two common causes of this lesion. (2 marks)

(b)   List three clinical signs you would expect to find. (3 marks)

(c)   Outline your investigations and further management. (4 marks)

Question 10

At a routine life assurance medical examination, a 47-year-old company director is found to have a blood pressure of 170/100. No other significant clinical abnormalities are noted.

(a) List four investigations you would perform. (2 marks)

(b) List four classes of drugs you may consider using in this case, with an example of each. (4 marks)

(c) Outline your management, assuming the diagnosis to be essential hypertension. (4 marks)

Question 11

A 27-year-old sales representative presents to her GP with a three-month history of worsening headaches, malaise and lethargy. On examination her blood pressure is found to be 190/100 both lying and standing. There are no other cardiovascular abnormalities noted.

(a) List three endocrine disorders, other than diabetes, that may present with hypertension. (3 marks)

(b) List three renal causes for hypertension. (3 marks)

(c) Outline your further investigations. (4 marks)

CHAPTER 7: HAEMATOLOGY

Question 1

A 37-year-old woman presents to her GP with a nine-month history of progressive lethargy and malaise now associated with exertional dyspnoea. On examination she is clinically anaemic, but no other abnormalities are detected. Routine blood tests reveal her to have a microcytic anaemia.

(a)   List three causes of a microcytic anaemia. (3 marks)

(b)   List the further investigations you would arrange. (3 marks)

(c)   List four gastrointestinal and four extra-intestinal causes for this woman's anaemia. (4 marks)

Question 2

A 63-year-old woman presents to the medical outpatient department with a one-year history of increasing lethargy, weight gain, and poor concentration. She also complains of dry hair and skin. Investigations confirm hypothyroidism and a macrocytic anaemia, with an MCV of 112 fl.

(a)   Give two causes for the raised MCV in this case. (2 marks)

(b)   Explain the autoimmune basis of her anaemia. (3 marks)

(c)   Briefly outline your further management. (5 marks)

Question 3

A 9-year-old boy with known sickle cell disease, presents to the Accident and Emergency department with a two-day history of an upper respiratory tract infection associated with pain in his ribs, back and hips. He also complains of severe left upper quadrant pain.

(a)   (i)   Name two other haemoglobinopathies. (2 marks)
       (ii)   What is the cause of his left upper quadrant pain? (1 mark)

(b)   Outline your therapeutic management in this case. (3 marks)

(c)   In each of the categories listed below, give one pathological change associated with sickle cell disease.
       (i) skin (ii) renal (iii) biliary tree (iv) bone. (4 marks)

Question 4

A 27-year-old man presents to his GP with a two-month history of weight loss, lethargy and night sweats, now associated with generalized pruritus. On examination he has generalized lymphadenopathy and hepatospleno-megaly. He denies any risk factors for HIV disease.

(a)   What is the diagnosis? (1 mark)

(b)   List five investigations to confirm the diagnosis. (5 marks)

(c)   Outline the therapeutic options. (4 marks)

Question 5

A 5-year-old girl presents to the paediatric outpatient department with a three-week history of nose bleeds and a purpuric rash following an upper respiratory tract infection. The results of a full blood count organised by her GP are Hb 13.2, WCC 7.8, platelets 31. The comment on the film reads 'no abnormal forms seen, grossly reduced platelet numbers'.

(a)   What is the likely cause of her thrombocytopaenia? (2 marks)

(b)   List five other causes. (5 marks)

(c)   Outline the therapeutic options in this case. (3 marks)

Question 6

A 6-year-old boy with known trisomy 21, presents to the paediatric outpatient department with a two-month history of malaise, lethargy and exertional dyspnoea, associated with easy bruising and several recent chest infections. On examination he has generalized lymphadenopathy and hepatosplenomegaly. He is clinically anaemic and has several large bruises.

(a)   What is the underlying diagnosis and why is it particularly relevant in this case? (2 marks)

(b)   List three investigations to confirm the diagnosis. (3 marks)

(c)   Briefly outline the management strategies used in this case. (5 marks)

Question 7

A 47-year-old woman presents to her GP with a two-month history of malaise, anorexia and an 8 kg weight loss, associated with left upper quadrant discomfort and occasional fever. On examination she is clinically anaemic and has a very enlarged spleen extending 15 cm below the left costal margin.

(a) (i) What is the likely haematological malignancy in this case? (1 mark)

  (ii) What is the chromosomal abnormality and the associated translocation? (1 mark)

(b) List two other causes of 'massive' splenomegaly. (2 marks)

(c) (i) List three essential investigations you would perform. (3 marks)

  (ii) Outline your management. (3 marks)

Question 8

A 62-year-old retired man presents to the Accident and Emergency department with a painful, bruised hip after a seemingly insignificant fall whilst out shopping. On examination he is clinically anaemic and has multiple bruises, particularly around his left hip, which is clinically fractured. This is confirmed on X-ray, which also reveals multiple lytic lesions throughout the pelvic and femoral bones.

(a)   State the descriptive term for this type of fracture and the underlying diagnosis. (2 marks)

(b)   List five investigations you would perform. (5 marks)

(c)   He has a corrected calcium of 4.2 mmol/l. Outline your treatment of this problem. (3 marks)

CHAPTER 8: DERMATOLOGY

Question 1

A 47-year-old obese woman presents to her GP with deep jaundice and intense pruritus, associated with moderate right upper quadrant pain which has been worsening over the last seven days.

(a)   What is the likely cause of her symptoms? (1 mark)

(b)   List four other disorders which may present with pruritus. (4 marks)

(c)   Outline the general principles for treating pruritus. (5 marks)

Question 2

A 16-year-old schoolgirl presents to the dermatology outpatient department with a two-week history of a red, tender, itchy rash over both palms, which coincided with her starting work at a hairdressers about one month before. In the past she has had a similar rash over the pinna of her ears, after having her ears pierced.

(a) (i) What is the name given to this type of rash? (2 marks)

 (ii) What is the likely cause in this case? (1 mark)

(b) List three other causes of this type of rash which may be relevant to this patient. (3 marks)

(c) Briefly outline your management of this patient. (4 marks)

Question 3

A 7-year-old boy with known atopic eczema is admitted to hospital with an acute exacerbation of his rash, with a 'weeping' area around the face which looks infected. He also has local areas of lichenification affecting knees, elbows and neck.

(a)   What does the term 'lichenification' mean? Which surfaces of the body does atopic eczema characteristically affect? (3 marks)

(b)   Give two disorders associated with atopic eczema. What is the immune mediated abnormality? (3 marks)

(c)   Outline your management in this case. (4 marks)

Question 4

A 29-year-old man with long standing psoriasis presents to his GP with a worsening psoriatic rash, which in areas demonstrates the Koebner phenomenon. The GP arranges for his admission to hospital.

(a)   What is the Koebner phenomenon? List two other disorders which demonstrate it. (3 marks)

(b)   List three sites, other than the extensor surfaces of the limbs, which may be affected by psoriasis. (3 marks)

(c)   List the therapeutic agents used in the treatment of psoriasis, giving a side effect of each. (4 marks)

Question 5

A 43-year-old woman presents to the Accident and Emergency department with a one-week history of a dry cough, fever and general malaise, now associated with a severe blistering rash over the hands and feet, and affecting her eyes and mouth. On examination blistering and 'target' lesions are seen, and coarse crackles are heard in both lung fields.

(a)   What is the name given to this rash and what is the eponymous syndrome which has developed? (2 marks)

(b)   What is the likely cause of the rash in this woman? List three other causes. (4 marks)

(c)   Outline your investigations and management. (4 marks)

Question 6

An 18-year-old woman presents to her GP with a seven-day history of fever, malaise and arthralgia associated with increasingly painful red, tender, round lesions over her shins. The symptoms have started since she began taking the oral contraceptive pill.

(a)   What is the lesion that has developed on her shins? (1 mark)

(b)   List four other causes of this lesion. (4 marks)

(c)   Briefly outline your management. (5 marks)

Question 7

A 72-year-old man presents to his GP with a blistering pruritic rash affecting his upper and lower limbs.

(a)   Give three causes of a blistering rash in a man of this age. (3 marks)

(b)   List three discerning questions you would ask in the history to differentiate the possible causes. (3 marks)

(c)   The rash displays Nikolsky's sign.
   (i)   What is this sign and what is the underlying diagnosis? (2 marks)
   (ii)   List two drugs used in its treatment. (2 marks)

Question 8

A 29-year-old ginger haired man presents to his GP with a new, large mole on his left upper arm. He has recently returned to the UK after living in South Africa for several years.

(a)   List the features that would concern you about this 'mole'. (4 marks)

(b)   List three skin conditions associated with excessive sunlight exposure. (3 marks)

(c)   What are the therapeutic options if this was found to be a malignant melanoma? (3 marks)

Question 9

A 46-year-old man is sent to dermatology outpatient department with 'abnormal nails'. On examination he has onycholysis.

(a)   Give two causes of onycholysis. (2 marks)

(b)   List two investigations for this patient. (2 marks)

(c)   What are the nail changes associated with the following disorders. (6 marks)
(i) Iron deficiency   (ii) Bronchiectasis   (iii) Infective endocarditis
(iv) Psoriasis   (v) Chemotherapy   (vi) Chronic liver disease

Question 10

Two teenage sisters are being investigated in the dermatology outpatient department for hair complaints. The older sister has a large well defined area of hair loss, her younger sister has excessive facial hair.

(a)   What are the medical terms given to these two conditions? (2 marks)

(b)   List two possible causes for each sister's problem. (4 marks)

(c)   Briefly outline your therapeutic management of the younger sister's complaint. (4 marks)

Question 11

A 37-year-old man presents to the dermatology outpatient department with areas of depigmentation over his hands and chest. A clinical diagnosis of vitiligo is made.

(a) List three disorders which may be associated with depigmentation. (3 marks)

(b) List three disorders which are associated with vitiligo. (3 marks)

(c) List the essential investigations you would perform. (4 marks)

CHAPTER 9: GASTROENTEROLOGY

Question 1

A 40-year-old man complains of progressive difficulty in swallowing solids with a recent onset of vomiting following meals.

(a)   How would you exclude a malignant stricture of the oesophagus? (3 marks)

(b)   Motility studies reveals abnormal peristalsis and sphincter spasm of the oesophagus.
   (i)   How is oesophageal function studied? (2 marks)
   (ii)   State the likely diagnosis and its underlying pathology. (2 marks)

(c)   How would you treat this condition? (3 marks)

Question 2

A 54-year-old woman presents with an 18-month history of heartburn, water brash and belching, with pain on swallowing.

(a)   State your diagnosis and the underlying mechanism. (3 marks)

(b)   How would you demonstrate acid reflux in this patient? (3 marks)

(c)   Outline the treatment of this condition. (4 marks)

Question 3

A 43-year-old male business executive is admitted through the Accident and Emergency department with a three-day history of vomiting 'coffee ground' material and 18 months of progressive dyspeptic symptoms, which are partially relieved by antacids.

(a)   State the probable clinical diagnosis. (2 marks)

(b)   State two investigations to confirm your diagnosis and the expected findings. (3 marks)

(c)   List the drugs and their therapeutic regimes used to cure this disease. (5 marks)

Question 4

A 36-year-old woman is referred to the gastroenterology clinic with a nine-month history of weakness and weight loss associated with intermittent abdominal discomfort and distension. The stools are bulky pale and greasy.

(a)   (i)   List three malabsorption states that would fit her symptoms. (3 marks)

        (ii)   State one investigation that would provide evidence for a definitive diagnosis, and list the possible findings. (2 marks)

(b)   The patient is placed on a gluten-free diet and obtains remission from her symptoms over the subsequent four months.

        (i)   State the likely diagnosis. (2 marks)

        (ii)   List the long-term complications of this condition. (3 marks)

Question 5

A 26-year-old woman is seen at the Accident and Emergency department with fever, malaise and bloody diarrhoea of six days' duration.

(a)   List the possible diagnoses from her presentation. (3 marks)

(b)   The patient is sent home on a course of antibiotics but her condition worsens, with abdominal pain and distension. She is febrile, with a pulse rate of 120/min. Sigmoidoscope examination reveals pus and blood with mucosal ulceration.
   (i)   State the diagnosis. (1 mark)
   (ii)   List three life-threatening complications that may ensue if treatment is further delayed. (3 marks)

(c)   How would you treat this patient? (3 marks)

Question 6

A 40-year-old woman with long-standing chronic bowel symptoms is diagnosed as having Crohn's disease.

(a) (i)   List the main symptoms of this disease. (2 marks)
     (ii) List four extra-gastrointestinal manifestations of this disease. (2 marks)

(b) List the medical measures used to treat an acute exacerbation of this disease. (3 marks)

(c) State the indications for surgery in this disease. (3 marks)

Question 7

A 30-year-old man known to have an AIDS-related illness complains of nausea, intermittent diarrhoea and crampy abdominal pain of increasing severity. Clinical examination is suggestive of subacute bowel obstruction.

(a) (i)   List two causes of bowel obstruction in AIDS. (2 marks)
     (ii) List three opportunistic organisms that cause enteric infection in AIDS. (3 marks)

(b) (i)   How would you confirm bowel obstruction in this patient? (2 marks)
     (ii) State the principles of treatment. (3 marks)

Question 8

A 29-year-old overseas visitor complains of malaise, abdominal pain and diarrhoea with the passage of blood-stained mucus over an eight-week period. A diagnosis of amoebic colitis is made on sigmoidoscopic examination.

(a) (i) List the characteristic sigmoidoscopic findings in this disease. (3 marks)

(ii) State how you would confirm the diagnosis. (2 marks)

(b) How would you screen for an amoebic liver abscess in this patient? (2 marks)

(c) List the drugs used to treat this disease. (3 marks)

Question 9

A **40-year-old male alcoholic presents with a 20-month history of progressive central abdominal pain, anorexia and weight loss, and habituation to analgesic drugs. There is no history of jaundice.**

(a)　(i)　State the probable clinical diagnosis. (1 mark)

　　　(ii)　State one blood test to confirm this. (1 mark)

(b)　His stools were bulky, pale and offensive, and his fasting blood sugar level was moderately elevated. State the causes for these findings. (3 marks)

(c)　How would you treat this patient? (5 marks)

Question 10

A 46-year-old man complains of anorexia, malaise and weakness and is found to have a palpably enlarged, firm and irregular liver. A clinical diagnosis of cirrhosis is made.

(a)   List other abdominal findings that are characteristic of this disease. (3 marks)

(b)   State four biochemical investigations used to assess the severity of this disease and their significance. (4 marks)

(c)   The patient subsequently has an episode of haematemesis. State its association with the underlying liver disease. (3 marks)

Question 11

A 42-year-old man with a history of alcohol abuse complains of anorexia, malaise and weight loss over a three-month period. On examination he is found to have an enlarged, tender liver.

(a)   Write a note on the clinical spectrum of alcoholic liver disease. (4 marks)

(b)   List the pathological features of the liver disease. (3 marks)

(c)   What are the prognostic indicators of this disease? (3 marks)

Question 12

Ten days after sustaining a severe head injury in a road traffic accident, a 26-year-old woman remains paralysed and ventilated in ITU. The nutrition team are asked to assess her with regard to her feeding requirements.

(a)   What are the two forms of feeding that may be used? (2 marks)

(b)   List four investigations or parameters that are used in the nutritional assessment. (4 marks)

(c)   List the factors which will determine what form of feeding you would recommend. (4 marks)

Question 13

A 39-year-old man, who is a known chronic alcohol abuser, is brought into the Accident and Emergency department in a state of haemodynamic shock. On arrival he vomits 500 ml of fresh blood.

(a)   (i)   What is the most likely cause of his haematemesis? (1 mark)

       (ii)   List four other causes. (2 marks)

(b)   List the essential blood tests you would perform. (3 marks)

(c)   Outline your management of this patient. (4 marks)

Question 14

A 66-year-old man is admitted as an emergency, having vomited a considerable quantity of blood at home and feeling weak and faint.

(a)　List the historical findings that may point to the cause of bleeding in the upper gastrointestinal tract. (4 marks)

(b)　State an investigation that provides an immediate diagnosis in this patient. (2 marks)

(c)　The cause of the bleeding is found to be an ulcerating tumour on the lesser curve of the stomach. List the investigations you would perform and state the definitive treatment. (4 marks)

CHAPTER 10: NEPHROLOGY

Question 1

A 27-year-old woman presents to the Accident and Emergency department with a two-day history of worsening left loin pain associated with fever, rigors and vomiting. It is her third such presentation in the past six months.

(a)   What is the diagnosis? (1 mark)

(b)   List four investigations you would perform on admission. (4 marks)

(c)   Briefly outline your further management. (5 marks)

Question 2

A 34-year-old woman is sent by her GP to the medical outpatient department with a three-month history of poorly controlled hypertension, recurrent UTI, and bilaterally palpable kidneys. A diagnosis of polycystic kidneys is confirmed on ultrasound scan.

(a)   Give two other causes of bilaterally enlarged kidneys. (2 marks)

(b)   List five complications of polycystic kidneys. (5 marks)

(c)   Outline the therapeutic management. (3 marks)

Question 3

A 15-year-old schoolboy presents to the Accident and Emergency department with a 10-day history of increasing ankle and leg oedema. He has felt lethargic but denies any other systemic symptoms or fever. Investigations reveal a nephrotic syndrome, secondary to minimal change nephropathy.

(a)   List the triad which characterizes a nephrotic syndrome. (3 marks)

(b)   List the electron microscopic changes that characterize minimal change nephropathy. (2 marks)

(c)   List three investigations you would perform, and outline your management of this patient. (5 marks)

Question 4

A 35-year-old man is admitted to the renal unit for investigation of a nephrotic syndrome secondary to a suspected glomerulonephritis.

(a) List three causes of a nephrotic syndrome. (3 marks)

(b) List three haematological and three non-haematological investigations you would perform. (5 marks)

(c) List two complications of the nephrotic syndrome. (2 marks)

Question 5

A 29-year-old woman who has had poorly controlled insulin-dependent diabetes mellitus for the past 15 years, presents to her GP with malaise and lethargy. She has recently been started on an ACE inhibitor for hypertension. Routine blood investigations arranged that day show:-
FBC: Hb 7.9, MCV 88, MCH 35, WCC 9.0, platelets 310
U+Es: Na 122, K 8.8, urea 37.1, creatinine 567

(a)   List two diagnoses that may be made from this data. (2 marks)

(b)   List three factors contributing to her deranged renal function. (3 marks)

(c)   Outline the management of hyperkalaemia. (5 marks)

Question 6

A 53-year-old woman with chronic rheumatoid arthritis is sent by her GP to the renal outpatient department with worsening renal impairment and signs suggestive of a nephrotic syndrome.

(a)   Give two possible causes of renal impairment in this patient. (2 marks)

(b)   List three non-haematological investigations you would perform. (3 marks)

(c)   Briefly outline your management of this patient. (5 marks)

Question 7

A 29-year-old man presents to the medical outpatient department with a three-week history of malaise, lethargy, arthralgia and myalgia, associated with a vasculitic rash. Examination reveals palpable nodules over several of his peripheral arteries and a blood pressure of 180/130. Routine urinalysis shows large amounts of protein and some blood.

(a)   What is the diagnosis? List two other causes of renal impairment and a vasculitic rash. (3 marks)

(b)   List two immune markers that may occur in this group of disorders. (2 marks)

(c)   List two other investigations you would perform, and outline your therapeutic management. (5 marks)

Question 8

A 39-year-old man presents to his GP with a four-month history of malaise and lethargy, but no other specific systemic symptoms. Routine blood investigations are: FBC: Hb 6.2, MCV 81, MCH 34, WCC 9.0, platelets 298; U+Es: Na 132, K 5.8, urea 45.7, creatinine 890, glucose 7.4, corrected calcium 1.76, phosphate 3.7; LFTs: albumin 18, AST 23, ALT 18, alkaline phosphatase 211.

(a)   List three features which indicate this man has chronic renal failure. (3 marks)

(b)   List three tests/investigations you could do in the GP surgery to elucidate the cause of his renal failure. (3 marks)

(c)   Briefly ouline your management of the
(i) anaemia (ii) renal impairment (iii) hypocalcaemia (iv) hyperphosphataemia. (4 marks)

Question 9

A 73-year-old woman is brought to the Accident and Emergency department by ambulance, after being found unconscious at home by a neighbour. On arrival she is confused, with a GCS of 12, and is haemodynamically stable. Initial investigations show: FBC: Hb 14.2, haematocrit 0.58, WCC 31.2 (neutrophilia), platelets 57; U+Es: Na 152, K 4.3, urea 35.7, creatinine 290, glucose 38.5 mmol/l.

(a)   List three diagnoses that can be inferred from these results. (3 marks)

(b)   List four further investigations you would perform. (4 marks)

(c)   List two causes of pre-renal, renal and post-renal impairment. (3 marks)

Question 10

A 5-year-old boy is admitted to hospital for investigation of a suspected renal tubular acidosis. Initial investigations by his GP show: U+Es: Na 134, K 3.1, chloride 114, bicarbonate 12, urea 4.1, creatinine 103.

(a)   Calculate the anion gap, showing your calculations. (3 marks)

(b)   List the three types of renal tubular acidosis, with a cause for each. (3 marks)

(c)   List two diabetic causes of a high anion gap acidosis, outlining the general principles of your therapeutic management. (4 marks)

CHAPTER 11: RHEUMATOLOGY AND CONNECTIVE TISSUE DISEASES

Question 1

A 29-year-old woman presents to the medical outpatient department with a four-month history of painful, swollen proximal interphalangeal joints, associated with early morning stiffness, malaise and lethargy. X-rays of her hands show a symmetrical erosive arthropathy affecting the proximal interphalangeal joints.

(a)   What is the likely cause of her arthropathy? (1 mark)

(b)   In the categories below, list an associated feature which may occur in this disorder: (i) eyes, (ii) skin, (iii) respiratory, (iv) cardiovascular, (v) renal. (5 marks)

(c)   Outline your therapeutic management of this patient. (4 marks)

Question 2

An obese 67-year-old woman presents to her GP with a four-month history of increasing swelling, pain and stiffness in her right knee. She suffered a comminuted fracture of the distal right femur in a car accident, 10 years previously.

(a)   What is the likely cause of her arthritis? (1 mark)

(b)   List the radiological features that you would expect on an X-ray of her right knee joint. (5 marks)

(c)   Briefly outline your therapeutic management of this patient. (4 marks)

Question 3

A 27-year-old woman presents in the rheumatology outpatient department, with a six-week history of malaise and lethargy associated with painful joints in her hands and a worsening rash over her cheeks. On examination the joints of her hands are tender but otherwise normal. There is a 'butterfly' rash over her cheeks and vasculitic changes around her finger nails.

(a)   What is the underlying diagnosis? (1 mark)

(b)   List three immune markers that may occur in this disorder. (3 marks)

(c)   In each of the categories below, list one pathological feature that may occur: (i) skin (ii) vascular (iii) renal (iv) neurological (v) haematological (vi) musculoskeletal. (6 marks)

Question 4

A 39-year-old woman presents to her GP with a one-year history of pain in her fingers and toes associated with 'blanching' on exposure to the cold. She also complains of tightness and swelling of the fingers and, more recently, dysphagia with solids.

(a)   What is the term used to describe the changes she experiences in the cold? (1 mark)

(b)   This disorder was previously called the CREST syndrome. What are the components of the syndrome and what is it called now? (4 marks)

(c)   Outline your therapeutic management of this patient. (5 marks)

Question 5

A 47-year-old man presents to his GP with an acutely hot, tender and swollen interphalangeal joint of his left big toe. He is otherwise systemically well.

(a)   What is the likely cause of his monoarthritis? (1 mark)

(b)   List three investigations to help confirm the diagnosis. (3 marks)

(c)   List three risk factors for developing this condition, and three drugs you might use in this man's treatment, with a side effect of each. (6 marks)

Question 6

A 71-year-old woman presents to her GP with a four-week history of stiffness and pain in her shoulders and thighs, particularly on waking in the morning. Routine investigations reveal an ESR of 105.

(a) What is the likely cause of her symptoms and the associated arteritis? (2 marks)

(b) Give two other musculoskeletal conditions that may cause an ESR over 100. (2 marks)

(c) With regard to the arteritis:
   (i) List one investigation to confirm the diagnosis. (2 marks)
   (ii) Which essential treatment must be instituted immediately? (1 mark)
   (iii) List three presenting symptoms. (3 marks)

Question 7

A 41-year-old man presents to the medical outpatient department with a six-month history of malaise and weight loss associated with a bloody nasal discharge, a chronic dry cough, episodic haemoptysis and exertional dyspnoea. On examination he has a vasculitic rash over his fingers and toes and coarse crackles are heard throughout both lung fields. Routine urinalysis shows large amounts of blood and protein in the urine.

(a)   State the diagnosis, and the classical triad which forms the basis of this diagnosis. (4 marks)

(b)   List two other causes of a vasculitic rash. (2 marks)

(c)   List three investigations you would perform, and name the drug that forms the basis of therapy. (4 marks)

Question 8

A 55-year-old woman, who had had a hysterectomy and bilateral salpingo-oophorectomy at the age of 34, presents to her GP with severe lumbar back pain. Routine blood tests are unremarkable, but X-rays of her lumbar spine show 'gross osteopaenia and vertebral collapse at L2/L3'.

(a)   What is the likely cause of her vertebral collapse? (1 mark)

(b)   (i)   List three risk factors for developing this condition. (3 marks)
       (ii)   List the therapeutic agents you would use in this case. (3 marks)

(c)   Outline the advice you would give her 22-year-old daughter with regard to prophylaxis. (3 marks)

Question 9

A 77-year-old man with known Paget's disease of the bone, presents to the Accident and Emergency department with a four-week history of increasing pain in his right hip and lumbar spine. He is now unable to bear weight.

(a)   What is the pathological basis of Paget's bone disease? (2 marks)

(b)   List three investigations you would perform to confirm the diagnosis. (3 marks)

(c)   List three complications of Paget's bone disease, and briefly outline your therapeutic management. (5 marks)

Question 10

A 63-year-old man with known ankylosing spondylitis presents to his GP with worsening mobility and lumbar back pain. On examination he has severely restricted lumbar and cervical spine movement and mild vertebral tenderness over the lumbosacral spine.

(a)   What is the HLA association of this disorder? List two other diseases that are linked to this HLA serotype. (3 marks)

(b)   List the radiological features that may be present on an X-ray of this man's lumbosacral spine. (3 marks)

(c)   In the categories below, list one pathological feature that may occur in this disorder.
(i) eyes, (ii) cardiac, (iii) respiratory, (iv) neurological. (4 marks)

Question 11

A 26-year-old man returns from a business trip in Bangkok with a one-week history of a painful urethral discharge associated with 'gritty', painful red eyes and a hot swollen left knee. In the last 24 hours he has also developed ulceration in his mouth and on the glans penis.

(a)   State the eponymous name given to the disorder described above, and the triad of symptoms which define it. (2 marks)

(b)   List three organisms that may precipitate it. (3 marks)

(c)   Briefly outline your investigations and therapeutic management. (5 marks)

CHAPTER 12: PSYCHIATRY

Question 1

A 39-year-old man reluctantly attends his GP with his wife. She feels that his alcohol intake is becoming a problem, but he can not see 'the harm of the odd drink here and there'.

(a)   What are the four elements of the CAGE questionnaire? (4 marks)

(b)   List two screening investigations to assess this man's alcohol intake. (2 marks)

(c)   Outline your management of this patient. (4 marks)

Question 2

A 72-year-old man, whose wife recently died in a road traffic accident, is found deeply unconscious in bed, by his neighbour. On the bedside table there is a long suicide note, accompanied by an empty bottle of pills.

(a)   List three features of the history that imply this was a serious suicide attempt. (3 marks)

(b)   List three other factors used to determine suicidal intent. (3 marks)

(c)   Briefly outline your management in this case. (4 marks)

Question 3

A 19-year-old student visits her college GP with a four-month history of amenorrhoea. She denies being pregnant and has put it down to the stress of the course. The GP can not help noticing that she is extremely thin, and on further questioning she does admit to eating 'very infrequently' recently.

(a)   What is the likely diagnosis? List two criteria used to make this diagnosis. (3 marks)

(b)   The student is 1.6 metres tall and weighs 30 kg. Calculate her BMI, showing your calculations. (3 marks)

(c)   List three investigations you would perform, and briefly outline your management. (4 marks)

Question 4

A 29-year-old known heroin addict is brought into to the Accident and Emergency department unconscious, with shallow respiration and a thready pulse.

(a)   (i)   What is the diagnosis, and the immediate management? (3 marks)

       (ii)   Which other physical sign will confirm the diagnosis? (1 mark)

(b)   List two routes of administration that are commonly used by heroin addicts. (2 marks)

(c)   In the categories below, list one symptom or sign that may be exhibited on the withdrawl of heroin.
(i) neurological, (ii) psychological, (iii) gastrointestinal, (iv) dermato-logical. (4 marks)

Question 5

A GP is called to see a 31-year-old woman, who has recently lost her 6-year-old daughter, who died of leukaemia. She has not been out since the funeral one month ago, and her husband is very worried that she has completely withdrawn into herself.

(a)   What is the underlying diagnosis? List two other features you would specifically try to elicit in the history. (3 marks)

(b)   List two non-pharmacological therapies that may be employed. (2 marks)

(c)   List the three main classes of antidepressants, with an example and a side effect of each class. (5 marks)

Question 6

A **26-year-old unemployed man is brought into the Accident and Emergency department by the police, who found him wandering naked in the local park. They say he was screaming at some men who were 'trying to kill him' when, in fact, he was alone. Examination and investigations are unremarkable and he is referred to the psychiatrist with a clinical diagnosis of schizophrenia.**

(a)   List two first rank symptoms of schizophrenia. (2 marks)

(b)   List two presenting and two premorbid features which indicate a poor prognosis in schizophrenia. (4 marks)

(c)   Briefly outline your therapeutic management. (4 marks)

Question 7

A 31-year-old man is brought to the psychiatric outpatient department by his wife, with a three-month history of working 20 hours per day whilst sleeping for only 2–3 hours. He claims he has become the managing director of his accountancy firm when, in fact, he has just been made redundant. She says he has also become sexually demanding. He was treated for depression by his GP one year previously.

(a) What are the terms used to describe his present condition and the underlying condition? (3 marks)

(b) List three presenting features of this disorder in the history. (3 marks)

(c) List two drugs used in the treatment of this disorder and a side effect of each. (4 marks)

Question 8

A 27-year-old man is referred by his lawyer to see a psychiatrist for assessment. He is a habitual criminal, with multiple convictions for violent crime. He has been married three times, each ending in divorce, after he was violent towards his family. He has never had a permanent job and is at present on remand, after fatally stabbing a man in a fight.

(a)   What is the term used to describe this man's behavioural disorder? (2 marks)

(b)   Define what is meant by a personality disorder, listing three other examples. (5 marks)

(c)   List the factors that may have influenced the development of this type of personality. (3 marks)

Question 9

A 32-year-old man is referred to the psychiatric outpatient department by his GP with a six-month history of washing his hands up to 50 times per day, to the point where his hands have become ulcerated and raw.

(a)   What is the term used to describe this condition? (2 marks)

(b)   Define the term neurosis, giving two examples. (4 marks)

(c)   Briefly outline your management. (4 marks)

CHAPTER 13: CARE OF THE ELDERLY

Question 1

A 77-year-old man presents in the outpatient department with his wife, who gives a six-month history of a stepwise progressive deterioration in his memory, associated with worsening confusion and urinary incontinence. He has had two previous strokes and has been hypertensive for the past 15 years.

(a)   What is the diagnosis? (1 mark)

(b)   List 10 questions you would use to assess the degree of this man's cognitive impairment. (5 marks)

(c)   List the important features you would elicit in the social history and the members of the multidisciplinary team you would employ to achieve plans to keep this man at home. (4 marks)

Question 2

An 83-year-old woman who is normally fit and well, is brought to the Accident and Emergency department, having being found lying confused on the bedroom floor by her neighbours. On examination, she has a GCS of 13, her BM is 28–44 and she is pyrexial with an axillary temperature of 38.0°C. She is in fast atrial fibrillation, and has coarse crackles at the right lung base. Her mental test score is 3/10, but there is no focal neurological deficit.

(a) Give one possible cause for her admission. (1 mark)

(b) List five haematological and five non-haematological investigations you would perform. (5 marks)

(c) Outline your therapeutic management. (4 marks)

Question 3

An 86-year-old woman presents to the outpatient department with a three-month history of recurrent falls. She is being treated with a loop diuretic and an ACEI for heart failure and low dose aspirin for ischaemic heart disease. She has recently been started on digoxin for atrial fibrillation.

(a)   Give three possible causes for this woman's falls. (3 marks)

(b)   List three investigations you would perform. (3 marks)

(c)   List a side effect of each of the medications she is taking. (4 marks)

Question 4

A 79-year-old woman with a three-year history of mild to moderate dementia presents to the outpatient department with a two-month history of worsening urinary incontinence.

(a)   List three possible causes for her incontinence. (3 marks)

(b)   List three investigations you would perform. (3 marks)

(c)   Outline the therapeutic options. (4 marks)

Question 5

An 81-year-old woman is recovering in hospital two weeks after sustaining a fractured right neck of femur. The orthopaedic surgeon has requested a review, to help with her recovery.

(a)   List three possible causes for her slow progress. (3 marks)

(b)   List six investigations you would request. (3 marks)

(c)   Outline your management plan for this woman's rehabilitation. (4 marks)

Question 6

An 84-year-old man is brought into the Accident and Emergency department by ambulance, after having been found unconscious at home. On examination he has a rectal temperature of 31°C, a GCS of 5, and a BM of 7–11. There is no focal neurological deficit, and he has flexor plantar responses. Cardiovascular examination reveals an irregular pulse, with a rate of 30 bpm, but the blood pressure is 110/70. The rest of the clinical examination is normal.

(a)   What is the cause of this man's coma? List three predisposing factors. (3 marks)

(b)   List six essential investigations you would perform. (3 marks)

(c)   Outline your management. (4 marks)

Question 7

A 91-year-old man is admitted to hospital with a three-month history of worsening prostatism, associated with lumbar back and rib pain. Subsequent investigation reveals him to have disseminated prostatic carcinoma with bony metastases.

(a) List the major symptoms you would address in this case. (3 marks)

(b) List six drugs that may be required in this man's treatment. (3 marks)

(c) Outline your management once the diagnosis has been confirmed. (4 marks)

SECTION II:
SAQ MODEL ANSWERS AND COMMENTS

CHAPTER 1: INFECTIOUS DISEASES ANSWERS

Answer 1   **Marks**

(a)   Chronic active hepatitis secondary to hepatitis B or C
       virus (HBV and HCV)   1

(b)   Transplacentally
       Blood borne –   sexual, blood transfusion, intravenous
                        drug abuse, tattooing   3

(c)   Investigations – hepatitis B and C serology
                         alpha fetoprotein
                         LFTs and clotting screen
                         US scan of the liver and liver biopsy

       Therapeutic management – consider interferon therapy
       Exclude the development of hepatocellular carcinoma
       Screen family members and sexual contacts   6

Comment

Viral hepatitis is a common cause of chronic liver disease, particularly in endemic areas such as South East Asia. It is the major aetiological risk factor in the development of primary hepatocellular carcinoma. HBV infection is caused by a DNA virus, which has three main antigenic components: the surface protein, HBs antigen, the core protein, HBc antigen, and a soluble protein produced from the core gene, HBe antigen. These all give rise to antibody responses, the significances of which are summarised below.

	Antigen	**Antibody**
HBs	Marker of viral replication, it is found in acute, chronic and carrier states.	Marker of immunity, it shows previous exposure to the virus or vaccination.
HBc	It is not usually seen in the blood and has no clinical significance.	There are two antibody responses, IgM and IgG. IgM is a marker of ongoing viral replication.
HBe	Marker of infectivity, its persistence in the plasma signifies a chronic or carrier state, with a high risk of infectivity.	This is a marker of low infectivity risk.

At-risk groups, such as health workers, should be vaccinated. Secondary prevention with hyperimmune serum globulin, containing antiHBs antibody, can also be given in cases of accidental exposure, e.g. needle stick injury. Antiviral treatment with alpha interferon is still under assessment in chronic active disease. It produces a 40% seroconversion in patients, from HBe antigen to HBe antibody positive. Paradoxically, those with the most serious derangement of liver architecture and function seem to show the best response to therapy. Other antiviral agents under investigation include vidarabine and tribavirin. In patients developing hepatocellular carcinoma, surgical resection or liver transplantation may be considered, although in localized disease, radiological embolization of the tumour now offers a less invasive approach. Chemotherapy using adriamycin is used as an adjunct.

Answer 2   **Marks**

(a)   Meningitis
        Neisseria meningitidis
        Streptococcus pneumoniae
        Haemophilus influenzae   3

(b)   Blood tests – FBC, U+Es, glucose
                      clotting screen to include D-dimer
                      and FDPs, blood cultures
        CT head scan – to exclude raised intracranial pressure
        Lumbar puncture – MC+S, protein, and glucose
        ASO titre
        Throat swab
        CXR   3

(c)   The patient should be nursed in a darkened, quiet room
        Intravenous access, IV fluids
        Analgesia and antiemetics
        Start empirical IV antibiotic therapy
        In children (<15 years old) dexamethasone
        Correction of clotting abnormalities using FFP and platelets
        Contact tracing and chemoprophylaxis   4

Comment
Bacterial meningitis remains a serious infection with a mortality of 10–50%, depending on the causative organism. It is essential therefore to have a low threshold of suspicion and to start empirical intravenous antibiotic treatment

whenever the diagnosis is being considered. The causative organisms tend to be age specific:

Neonates: *E. coli*, Listeria, Group B Streptococci

Children (<15): *Neisseria meningitidis, Streptococcus pneumoniae, Haemophilus influenzae*

Adults: similar to children but also *Staphylococcus aureus, E. coli* and Listeria

If delays are envisaged at any point in the management then empirical IV antibiotic therapy should be given using benzylpenicillin, cefotaxime, ceftazidine, or ceftriaxone. Chloramphenicol is still used in some cases, but it is highly toxic and must be used with caution. In children under the age of 15, intravenous or oral dexamethasone should be given, as this reduces the post-meningitic complications, in particular deafness and residual cerebral damage. Symptomatic relief with appropriate analgesia, intravenous fluids and anti-emetics are important in all cases. In severe cases with septicaemic shock, DIC, and multi-organ failure the patient will require intensive care with inotrope support and occasionally, renal dialysis.

Answer 3   Marks

(a)   *Mycobacterium tuberculosis*   1

(b)   Blood cultures – MC+S, AAFBs
        Sputum for MC+S, AAFBs
        Stool culture
        CXR
        Barium meal and follow-through
        Laparoscopic biopsy of affected bowel   5

(c)   Rifampicin – derangement of LFTs, causes secretions,
                e.g. urine, to turn red
        Isoniazid – peripheral neuropathy (therefore given with
                pyridoxine)
        Pyrizinamide – hepatotoxic
        Streptomycin – ototoxic
        Ethambutol – optic neuritis   4

Comment

This woman has developed disseminated tuberculosis infection (TB), involving the lungs and terminal ileum. Diagnosis may be inferred by chest X-ray and barium follow-through appearances, and confirmed by the presence of alcohol and acid fast bacilli (AAFB) in sputum, blood and biopsy specimens. In cases where the small bowel is affected the patient may present with a clinical picture similar to that of terminal ileal Crohn's disease. However, this is rare in people of the Indian subcontinent and an empirical trial of antituberculous treatment should be started. As in any disorder presenting with chronic diarrhoea, a full nutritional assessment of the patient should be made, and possible nutritional support instituted. Management of any patient with tuberculosis should include a full course of antituberculous treatment, and contact tracing. Those in close contact with the patient should be tested for the disease by Mantoux testing and chest X-ray. Those tested negative should then receive BCG inoculation. Patients should receive regular follow up to ensure compliance and treatment success, as well as patient wellbeing. Ideally this should be directed from a centre and team dedicated to tuberculosis treatment. Non-compliance has lead to the emergence of resistant strains of tuberculosis (MDRTB), particularly in the USA. Most patients in the UK are placed on the regimes shown below:

- Pulmonary disease – 2 months – rifampicin, isoniazid, pyridoxine and pyrizinamide; 4 months – rifampicin and isoniazid (streptomycin and ethambutol are reserved for resistant cases)

In TB meningitis and disseminated disease, the regime is given for one year, with each period above being doubled.

Answer 4   **Marks**

(a)   *Plasmodium vivax, Plasmodium ovale* – chloroquine and
          primaquine
      Plasmodium falciparum – quinine and fansidar
      Plasmodium malariae   3

(b)   Blood tests – FBC, U+Es, glucose, LFTs, clotting screen
      Thick and thin blood films for malaria
      Blood cultures
      MSU
      CXR
      Stool cultures for ovum, parasites and cysts   3

(c)   Primary prophylaxis against being bitten by mosquitos
      Mosquito net over the bed, mosquito repellant, wear pyjama
      trousers and sleeves at night

Full course of antimalarial tablets, stressing the need for full
compliance
Ensure all vaccinations, including typhoid, tetanus, polio,
hepatitis A and B, are up to date   4

Comment

Malaria remains one of the commonest infectious causes of mortality worldwide, accounting for over a million deaths per year. It is endemic in Central
and South America, sub-Saharan Africa, the Middle East, the Indian sub-
continent, and South East Asia. In these areas, there is a high prevalence of
haemoglobinopathies amongst the local population and this confers a natural
resistance to the disease. So-called 'benign' malaria is caused by three species
of the parasite, *Plasmodium vivax*, *Plasmodium ovale* and *Plasmodium
malariae*. Although they tend to run a benign course, these parasites are
responsible for chronic disease due to the dormant hepatic phase in their life
cycle. This varies between months and years, and gives rise to hepatomegaly,
'giant' splenomegaly and chronic renal failure. They are invariably sensitive
to chloroquine, (reported resistance is limited principally to Papua New
Guinea), and if identified in blood films, the hepatic phase should be covered
for with primaquine. Falciparum malaria is termed the 'malignant' malaria,
and is responsible for the majority of the associated mortality. Death is caused
by cerebral involvement, DIC and multiorgan failure. There may be acute
renal tubular necrosis or a glomerulonephritis causing renal failure and,
commonly, there is pulmonary oedema and secondary bronchopneumonia,
which is often the terminal event. In all cases of suspected malaria, falciparum
disease must always be covered for, until there is definite species
identification. The patient should be started immediately on quinine either
orally, or, if severely unwell or cerebral involvement is suspected,
intravenously. Other drugs used in the treatment of falciparum disease include
fansidar and halofantrine.

Answer 5   **Marks**

(a) Infectious mononucleosis caused by the Epstein–Barr
     virus (EBV)
     Cytomegalovirus (CMV)
     Toxoplasmosis
     HIV
     Lymphoma   3

(b) FBC with differential, blood film and monospot test
Paul–Bunnell test
Specific antibody tests for EBV, CMV, toxoplasmosis
Throat swab
ASO titre
Lymph node biopsy   5

(c) Most of the causes are self-limiting, requiring symptomatic
relief only, i.e. analgesia for the pharyngitis, regular
paracetamol for pyrexia and fluids
Severe cases may require hospitalization and specific
treatment, e.g. steroids in EBV infection   2

Comment

EBV, CMV and toxoplasmosis may all present in a similar clinical manner, with pharyngitis, lymphadenopathy and splenomegaly associated with a low grade fever and flu-like symptoms. Infectious mononucleosis is caused by the Epstein–Barr virus and most commonly presents in adolescents and young adults. It is usually a self-limiting disorder, requiring no specific treatment. In more severe cases the use of steroids is advocated. Common sequelae include:

- Meningitis, encephalitis
- Myocarditis
- Hepatitis
- Splenomegaly – more rarely splenic rupture
- Guillain–Barré syndrome
- Haemolytic anaemia and thrombocytopaenia

EBV infection is strongly linked to the development of Burkitt's lymphoma. CMV infection is particularly prevalent in immunocompromized patients, being common in HIV positive and transplant patients. In these patients it may produce a severe illness, similar to EBV infection and should be treated with intravenous ganciclovir. It is differentiated from EBV infection by specific IgG and IgM antibodies, and the presence of intranuclear 'owl eyes' inclusions in tissue biopsies. Toxoplasmosis is a protozoan infection, caused by *Toxoplasma gondii*. Humans act as the intermediate host in its life cycle. The infection is usually carried by cats which are infected by killing and eating infected mice and birds. It is usually a self-limiting disorder, but may present in the immunocompromized as a severe febrile illness, involving the liver, spleen, central nervous system and heart. This is treated with a combination of pyrimethamine and sulphadiazine. Steroids are used in occular disease. The infection may also be acquired transplacentally, where it produces a chronic central nervous system disorder, characterized by hydrocephalus, cerebral calcification, chorioretinitis and seizures, classically known as the syndrome of Savin.

Answer 6   **Marks**

(a)   Pulmonary or oesophageal candidiasis
        Toxoplasmosis or CMV involving the central nervous system
        Pneumocystis carinii pneumonia (PCP)
        Kaposi's sarcoma (under 60 years old)   3

(b)   Cerebral abscess secondary to toxoplasmosis
        Lymphoma
        Primary brain tumour   2

(c)   FBC, differential and CD4 count
        U+Es
        Glucose
        Blood cultures
        CXR
        CT head scan with contrast
        Consider lumbar puncture and brain biopsy   5

Comment
Acquired immunodeficiency syndrome (AIDS) is caused by the retrovirus HTLV III (human T-lymphotropic virus III), also known as human immuno-deficiency virus, HIV I. A different form of the virus, HIV II, has been discovered more recently, and is the principal cause of HIV infection in Western Africa. There are several stages of HIV infection prior to the development of AIDS. Acute infection with the virus may be asymptomatic or may present with an acute seroconversion illness, similar to infectious mononucleosis. Persistent generalized lymphadenopathy (PGL) may be another acute presentation. There then follows a chronic phase, which has variable progression dependent on the HIV infection and possible genetic and other infectious co-factors.

The chronic phase is divided into an early, intermediate and late phase by clinical manifestations of the infection and various immune markers. Combinations of the various clinical signs and symptoms in the late phase are termed the AIDS related complex, or ARC.

Markers which define likely progression to AIDS include:
- Falling CD4 count – once below 400 cells/microlitre, opportunistic infections are increasingly likely. A count significantly below 400, with a decreased CD4:CD8 ratio, are poor prognostic indicators.
- Low or falling P24 antibody levels – P24 is a core protein expressed by HIV.
- Rising P24 levels indicate an acute viraemia, and when associated with low or falling P24 antibody level indicates an early predisposition to AIDS.

Other markers include – pancytopaenia, raised ESR and raised beta-2-microglobulin and IgA levels. AIDS defining illnesses are shown below:
- Infective – disseminated atypical mycobacterium infection; cerebral toxoplasmosis or CMV; pulmonary or oesophageal candidiasis; *Pneumocystis carinii* pneumonia, (PCP); cryptosporidium-related diarrhoea lasting longer than one month; extra-pulmonary cryptococcosis; herpes simplex infection pulmonary, oesophageal or mucocutaneous, for longer than one month; HIV encephalopathy
- Non-infective – cerebral lymphoma or Kaposi's sarcoma – below 60 years old; progressive multifocal leucoencephalopathy

Answer 7 **Marks**

(a) (i) Chancre of primary syphilis or gonorrhoea   1
     (ii) *Neisseria gonorrhoeae*
          Treponema pallidum   2

(b)   Other sexually acquired infections – HBV and HCV infection
      HIV
      Chlamydial NSU
      Genital and oral HSV infection
      Anal and genital warts   3

(c)   Urethral swab – MC+S, wet preparation for trichomonas
      Syphilis serology
      HIV test, with pre-test counselling
      Treatment – procaine penicillin by intramuscular injection
      If allergic to penicillin – tetracycline or erythromycin
      Tracing of sexual contacts
      Education about sexual behaviour   4

Chapter 1: Infectious Diseases Answers

Comment

Syphilis is a sexually transmitted disease, caused by the spirochaete *Treponema pallidum*. Except for a slight rise in the early 1970s, its incidence has continued to fall throughout the 20th century, principally as a result of effective antibiotic therapy. It is divided into primary, secondary and tertiary infection by various clinical manifestations. The duration of each phase varies between weeks and years. Syphilis serological tests indicate the stage and infectivity of the disease, and are explained below.

	VDRL	TPHA	FTA
Primary – early	–	–	+
Primary – late	+	+	+
Secondary	rising titres	+	+
Tertiary	rising titres	+	+

The *Treponema pallidum* haemagglutination assay (TPHA), and the fluorescent treponema antibodies–absorbed test (FTA), are highly specific markers of syphilitic infection, but they will always remain positive once exposure has occurred. They therefore cannot be used to diagnose reinfection.

The venereal disease research laboratory test (VDRL), usually becomes positive 4–6 weeks after an initial exposure, but will return to negative again after approximately 6 months. Rising VDRL titres are therefore used to monitor acute reinfections. False positive VDRL results occur with several conditions, shown below. The levels in these disorders, however, are usually lower than 1:8.

- False positive VDRL – infection (tuberculosis, malaria,viral hepatitis, EBV); mycoplasma; malignancy; chronic liver disease; connective tissue disorders; old age

Answer 8   Marks

(a) (i) Acute gastroenteritis   1

(ii) *Salmonella enteritidis*
Campylobacter jejuni
Enterotoxigenic *E. coli*   3

(b) Foreign travel
Contact with person exhibiting similar symptoms
– both by faecal–oral cross infection   2

(c)   Investigations –   FBC, U+Es, glucose, LFTs
                                          Blood cultures
                                          Stool cultures
                                          Plain AXR

Most cases are self-limiting and do not require any specific treatment

More severe cases – Admit and isolate if possible
                                    Supportive treatment with analgesia,
                                    IV fluids and antiemetics
                                    Antibiotic therapy may be appropriate
                                        when specific organisms are
                                        identified, e.g. salmonella
                                    Tracing of contacts and food source   4

Comment

Gastroenteritis is a group of usually self-limiting disorders, characterized by diarrhoea and vomiting. They are spread through faecal–oral contamination, principally through contaminated water and foods. The onset of symptoms usually gives some indication of the causative organism, and it is therefore essential to try and obtain a clear history from the patient. For example, vomiting 4–6 hours after a meal is suggestive of toxin-producing *Staphylococcus aureus* infection, or *Bacillus cereus*. Pathogenicity is usually through one of two main mechanisms. *Vibrio cholerae*, enterotoxigenic *E. coli*, and *Staphylococcus aureus* mediate their effects through toxin production. Salmonella, shigella, rotavirus and campylobacter cause mucosal damage with or without direct invasion. Most gastroenteritis requires only supportive treatment, i.e. maintaining adequate hydration, antiemetics and analgesia, if necessary. More serious cases, with a generalized systemic illness, require admission, isolation, and treatment with antibiotics. Most organisms are sensitive to metronidazole or ciprofloxacin.

In patients where salmonella and *E. coli* species are isolated, contact tracing should be organized, particularly if the source is thought to be a cafe, restaurant, butcher, or cooked meat suppliers, as these are notifiable illnesses in the UK.

Answer 9   **Marks**

(a) (i) Septic or septicaemic shock   1
     (ii) Urinary tract infection secondary to the catheter
             Intravenous cannula site infection
             Post-operative chest infection   3

(b)   FBC, U+Es, glucose
Clotting screen to include D-dimer and FDPs
Group and save
Blood cultures
Urine cultures
CXR
ECG
ABGs
Wound swab
Cannulae and catheter replaced and tips sent for culture;
swab of cannulae sites   3

(c)   Rapid assessment of the patient, trying to ascertain the
           cause of shock, i.e. sepsis site, myocardial infarction,
           gastrointestinal bleed, pulmonary embolism
Lie the patient flat if possible, with the foot of the bed
           raised
In this case – resite intravenous access
                 consider central venous line
                 start colloid infusion
                 broad spectrum antibiotics
                 oxygen via face mask
                 call senior colleague to assess   3

Comment

Septicaemic shock in hospitalized patients is commonly associated with Gram-negative organisms from the urinary, gastrointestinal or biliary tract. Other causative organisms include *Streptococcus pneumoniae*, *Staphylococcus aureus* and *Staphylococcus epidermidis*. Prognosis is principally influenced by the patient's premorbid state and evidence of multiorgan involvement or failure. The presence of a normal or subnormal body temperature indicates a very poor prognosis. The condition continues to have significant associated mortality, particularly at the extremes of life. Various cytokines and leucotrienes are responsible for the inflammatory response to the infecting organisms which, in turn, cause shock and secondary multi-organ failure. It is hoped that by manipulation of these mediators the prognosis will eventually be improved.

Answer 10   **Marks**

(a)   Amoebiasis with liver abscess
        Entamoeba histolytica   2

(b)   Liver abscess, which has caused hepatic enlargement,
        diaphragmatic irritation and referred shoulder pain   2

(c) (i) FBC, LFTs and clotting screen
        Stool culture – microscopy for ovum, cysts and parasites
        Proctoscopy and rectal biopsy
        Ultrasound scan of the liver
        Ultrasound guided aspiration of abscess – contents sent for
        MC+S   3

    (ii) Treatment – isolate the patient, supportive treatment –
                        rehydration
                        nutritional support
                        analgesia for hepatic and shoulder pain
        Antibiotics, e.g. metronidazole
        Followed by percutaneous aspiration of abscess under
        ultrasound or CT guidance   3

Comment

Amoebiasis may be divided into two forms. The non-invasive, asymptomatic form is characterized only by cyst excretion in the stool, and causes no associated mucosal pathology. The invasive form presents with an acute infective colitis, characterized by bloody diarrhoea and 'flask' shaped ulcers within the mucosa. The colitis may be limited to a small area or present as a pancolitis. Haematogenous spread after mucosal invasion may cause hepatic abscess formation. This initially gives few systemic symptoms, but with enlargement progresses to cause swinging pyrexia, rigors, and right upper quadrant pain. Diagnosis is confirmed by amoebic cysts in the stool, specific serological markers for amoebiasis and rectal or colonic biopsies. Hepatic involvement is demonstrated on ultrasound or CT scan, and is confirmed by cysts in the aspirated material. Treatment is principally medical with 75–80% of cases responding to metronidazole or tinidazole. Diloxanide furoate is often given after the initial course of antibiotics to kill any remaining cysts within the colonic lumen. Slowly regressing abscesses are aspirated percutaneously under imaging, surgical drainage being rarely required. Complications of amoebiasis include colonic perforation, rupture of hepatic abscesses and extension of abscesses into the pleural and pericardial spaces, which require immediate drainage.

Answer 11   Marks

(a) (i) Parasitic worm infestation, e.g. strongyloides, filariasis,

hookworm, roundworm	1
(ii) Drug hypersensitivity and allergic disorders	
Asthma and polyarteritis nodosa	2

(b)   The respiratory symptoms are due to pulmonary eosinophilia 2

(c)   FBC with differential and blood film
U+Es, LFTs, glucose, calcium and phosphate, B12 and folate
Specific serological markers for parasitic worms
CXR
Stool culture
Duodenal aspirate via endoscopy   5

Therapy is directed at the specific causative organism. Mebendazole, thiobendazole, albendazole and diethyl carbamazine are commonly used.

Comment

Parasitic worm infestations are common in tropical areas. They may present with malabsorption and weight loss and can produce a pulmonary eosinophilia, with asthma-like symptoms. Malabsorption may be confirmed on routine investigations by a raised MCV, low B12 and folate, low albumin and calcium. Infestation is confirmed by the presence of specific serological markers to the various organisms, isolation in stool cultures and duodenal aspirate. Pulmonary eosinophilia is the association of a peripheral eosinophilia with respiratory symptoms, such as dry cough and wheeze. The acute form is usually secondary to parasitic infection or drugs, e.g. NSAIDs or antibiotics. With continuing exposure this may develop into a chronic disorder. Other pulmonary conditions may present in this manner, e.g. asthma, polyarteritis nodosa and extrinsic allergic alveolitis. Other causes of eosinophilia include idiopathic hypereosinophilic syndrome, and haematological malignancies such as CML and lymphoma.

Answer 12	**Marks**

(a) (i) A fungus	1
(ii) Candidiasis – oropharyngeal and vaginal	
Ringworm infection – *Trichophyton rubrum*	
Athletes foot – *tinea pedis*	2

(b)   CXR
        Histoplasma antibody titres
        Blood cultures
        Sputum culture
        In severe cases – bone marrow aspirate for MC+S   3

(c)   Amphotericin – nephrotoxic, hepatotoxic and cardiotoxic
        Fluconazole – diarrhoea, Stevens–Johnson syndrome
        Griseofulvin – peripheral neuropathy, photosensitivity,
              enzyme inducer
        Itraconazole – peripheral neuropathy, cholestatic jaundice
        Ketoconazole – hepatitis, gynaecomastia
        Nystatin – rashes, diarrhoea
        Terbinafine – diarrhoea, Stevens–Johnson syndrome   4

Comment

Histoplasmosis is a fungal infection, which has two clinical forms, classical and African. Classical infection is caused by *Histoplasma capsulatum* which is found in the soil of endemic areas such as Australasia, South East Asia and the southern states of America. Its growth is particularly facilitated by the presence of bird excreta and bat guano, and therefore it is commonly found in caves where bats are nesting and around chicken farms. The infection may be divided into three main forms:

* asymptomatic exposure and sensitization – this accounts for 99% of cases
* pulmonary disease
* generalized systemic infection.

Acute pulmonary disease occurs 2–3 weeks after an initial exposure, e.g. on a caving holiday. It presents with fever, malaise, and a non-productive cough, classically associated with erythema nodosum, and a flitting arthritis. Radiologically, the chest X-ray changes are often florid compared to the clinical condition of the patient, and there may be diffuse patchy shadowing and bilateral hilar lymphadenopathy. Usually only supportive treatment is necessary, but in more severe cases with associated hypoxia, intravenous antifungal agents are required.

Chronic pulmonary disease is principally seen in endemic areas, arising due to chronic exposure. It is particularly prevalent in male smokers with underlying airways disease. The resulting disease leads to pulmonary cavitation and fibrosis, and patients require antifungal therapy and, in more advanced cases, lobectomy.

Generalized systemic disease is principally seen at the extremes of life and in immunocompromized patients. It commonly affects the liver, spleen and bone marrow, but may also infiltrate the gut, central nervous system, and rarely the heart, causing endocarditis. The diagnosis is made by bone marrow and sputum culture and positive complement-fixing antibodies. Treatment is with intravenous itraconazole or amphotericin.

CHAPTER 2: METABOLIC DISEASES ANSWERS

Answer 1   **Marks**

(a)   Kayser–Fleischer rings
      Copper (Cu)   2

(b)   LFTs and clotting
      Liver biopsy
      Serum caeruloplasmin
      Urinary copper   3

(c)   D-penicillamine
      Low copper diet
      Consider liver transplant
      Genetic counselling and family screening   5

Comment

Wilson's disease (hepatolenticular degeneration) is an autosomal recessive disorder, the abnormal gene having been isolated to chromosome 13. The disorder arises due to defective metabolism of copper within the biliary tree, causing its deposition in various sites around the body. The principal sites affected are:

- **Liver** – the disease in its early stages produces mild hepatic dysfunction, but with progression produces cirrhosis with portal hypertension and oesophageal varices. Some patients present with chronic active hepatitis, which may conceal the underlying diagnosis.
- **Central nervous system** – classically the disease produces an extra-pyramidal movement disorder, with tremor, chorea and facial grimacing. Other presentations include dysarthria, dysphasia and Parkinsonism. Frank psychiatric symptoms may also occur but are usually in association with neurological symptoms and signs.
- **Eyes** – the Kayser–Fleischer rings are due to copper deposition in Descemet's membrane of the cornea. They appear grey in dark eyes and brown in light coloured eyes.
- **Kidneys** – the disease is associated with an acquired Fanconi's syndrome, producing a type II (proximal) or a type IV (distal) renal tubular acidosis, depending on the site of predominant damage.
- **Cardiac** – deposition of copper in the myocardium produces a cardio-myopathy and results in biventricular cardiac failure.

- **Skin and joints** – the skin becomes a pigmented grey colour, whereas the joints may be hypermobile and premature osteoarthritis of the spine is common. Patients may develop a polyarthritis.

Treatment is dependent on early recognition of the disease, and implementation of the chelating agent, D-penicillamine. Liver transplant is potentially curative.

Answer 2   **Marks**

(a) Haemochromatosis
Accumulation of iron (Fe) in the body   3

(b) FBC, glucose, LFTs, clotting
Serum Fe, ferritin, TIBC
USS of the liver and pancreas
Liver biopsy   4

(c) (i) Pancreatic infiltration leading to diabetes mellitus
(ii) Melanin deposition in the skin
(iii) Pyrophosphate arthropathy   3

Comment
Primary haemochromatosis is an idiopathic disorder of iron metabolism, which is inherited in an autosomal recessive manner. The disorder leads to iron overload and deposition in various organs, including the liver, pancreas, and the myocardium, causing cirrhosis, diabetes mellitus and a cardiomyopathy. The classical bronzed appearance is due to melanin deposition not iron. The diagnosis is confirmed by a raised serum iron and a greatly increased saturation of the TIBC and serum ferritin. The liver disease is confirmed by biopsy. Treatment is aimed at lowering the iron level by regular venesection, which is performed at least once a week. Early detection and family screening dramatically improves the prognosis. Acquired iron overload, haemosiderosis, is most commonly seen in patients receiving repeated transfusions for chronic haemolytic diseases, particularly beta thalassaemia. The iron overload results from the transfusions and increased iron release. In these patients desferrioxamine may be used to chelate the excess iron.

Answer 3   **Marks**

(a)   Familial hypercholesterolaemia
        (Fredrickson hyperlipidaemia type IIa)
        Autosomal dominant   2

(b)   Signs –   corneal arcus
                        tendon xanthoma
                        periorbital xanthoma
        Bedside tests –   BM stix measurement, blood pressure,
                                urinalysis for glycosuria   4

(c)   Address all other risk factors for atherosclerotic disease, i.e.
                smoking, alcohol excess, obesity, hypertension, diabetes
                mellitus
        Dietitian review – strict low fat diet
        Medical treatment – initially a member of the statin group of
                lipid lowering agents, e.g. simvostatin
        Arrange sibling and family screening   4

Comment

Familial hypercholesterolaemia is a common inherited disorder of lipid
metabolism which is particularly prevalent in the UK and North America. It
is caused by defective LDL catabolism, resulting in an increase in LDL
cholesterol. Patients' cholesterol is usually in the range of 8–11 mmol/1. More
uncommonly it is also associated with an increase in VLDL, which causes an
associated hypertriglyceridaemia. Patients present with symptoms of premature atherosclerotic disease, i.e. IHD, CVAs and peripheral vascular
disease. Hyperlipidaemia is classified by the Fredrickson/WHO classification,
as shown below:-

Type	Lipoprotein increased	Lipid increased
I	Chylomicrons	Triglycerides (TGs)
IIa	LDL	Cholesterol
IIb	VLDL and LDL	TGs and cholesterol
III	Beta VLDL	TGS and cholesterol
	(IDL and chylomicron remant)	

In the mixed hyperlipidaemias, the fibrate group of drugs is preferred to the
statins, as they lower both cholesterol and triglyceride levels more effectively.

Answer 4   **Marks**

(a)   The glycogen storage diseases   2

(b)   Autosomal recessive
      Wilson's disease
      Haemochromatosis
      Sickle cell disease
      Thalassaemia
      Infantile polycystic kidney disease   4

(c)   Obtain a clear history from the parents, particularly a
      family history
      Examination – short stature, obesity, hepatomegaly
      Investigations –   FBC, U+Es including bicarbonate,
                              glucose, LFTs, clotting
                              Urinalysis
                              USS of liver and kidneys
                              Liver or renal biopsy for histological
                              diagnosis   4

Comment

The glycogen storage diseases are a rare group of disorders, caused by various enzyme defects in the metabolism or catabolism of glycogen. They therefore present with signs and symptoms of dysfunction of the two principal sites of glycogen utilization, the liver and the skeletal muscle. They all share common features and present in the neonate or the first two years of life.

Those that mainly affect the liver, such as glucose-6-phosphatase deficiency (Von Gierke's disease), present with hepatomegaly, growth retardation and obesity. Von Gierke's disease classically presents with a bleeding tendency, as there is an acquired Von Willebrand-like defect of the platelets, and attacks of hypoglycaemia and lactic acidosis. The diagnosis is confirmed by liver biopsy and specific histochemical staining. Treatment is aimed at maintaining normoglycaemia, which is achieved by overnight nasogastric glucose supplementation. This avoids the complications of hyperuricaemia and gout, hyperlipidaemia and acidosis, which in turn promote normal growth and a much improved prognosis. Without such treatment the patient develops increasing hepatic and renal dysfunction, leading to premature death. These patients are at risk of developing hepatocellular carcinoma. Disorders principally affecting the musculature, e.g. Pompe's disease, present with a generalized defect of cardiac and skeletal muscle, with associated hepatic abnormalities. They carry a poor prognosis and the patients do not survive beyond the age of 1 or 2 years. There is no specific treatment.

Answer 5   **Marks**

(a) Sweating, palpitations and pyrexia
     Motor weakness
     Mania, depression, hallucination   2

(b) Drugs, e.g. benzodiazepines
     Acute infection
     Prolonged fasting
     Oestrogen and progesterone, e.g. pregnancy and the oral
     contraceptive pill   3

(c) Acute –   analgesia (opiates)
                 remove the precipitating factor
                 propranolol for symptoms of sympathetic
                     overactivity
                 haematin therapy
                 ensure adequate carbohydrate intake
                 if signs of motor neuropathy – consider ITU
                     for assisted ventilation   5
     Prevention – education of the patient with regard to possible
                 precipitating factors

Comment

The porphyrias are a group of disorders which arise due to various enzyme defects in the haem synthesis pathway. They are divided into acute and non-acute porphyrias. The acute porphyrias, acute intermittent, variegate and hereditary coproporhyria, are characterized by acute attacks, triggered by environmental agents. Acute intermittent porphyria is the commonest, and is inherited in an autosomal dominant manner. It is five times more common in women, principally due to oestrogen hormones in the oral contraceptive pill and during pregnancy. Biochemically they are characterized by an excess of urinary porphobilinogen and delta aminolaevulinic acid. Clinically the patient may present with severe abdominal pain and vomiting, which may resemble an acute abdomen. The other acute porphyrias may also present with a photosensitive rash, due to excess porphyrin production. Drugs are a common precipitating factor in the acute presentations. Drugs that may cause an acute attack include: tricyclic antidepressants and MAOIs; barbiturates and benzodiazepines; antibiotics, sulphonamides and cephalosporins; diuretics and sulphonylureas. The non-acute porphyrias are *porphyria cutanea tarda*, congenital porphyria and erythropoietic protoporphyria. *Porphyria cutanea tarda* is characterized by a photosensitive bullous rash which produces scarring on healing. It may be precipitated by alcohol, and is associated with mild iron overload which leads to chronic liver disease. Treatment includes regular venesection and chloroquine, which increases urinary excretion of uroporphyrin. Congenital porphyria is a rare autosomal recessive disorder producing a severe photosensitive bullous rash which causes disfiguring scarring. Erythropoietic protoporphyria is an autosomal dominant disorder which produces pain and discolouration of the skin on exposure to sunlight, associated with chronic liver disease. Treatment with beta carotene improves the skin condition.

Answer 6   **Marks**

(a) Tay–Sach's disease
     Inflammatory bowel disease   2

(b) (i) Sphingolipidoses
        Autosomal recessive   2
   (ii) FBC
        Clotting screen
        LFTs
        USS of the liver and spleen   3

(c) There is a relatively good prognosis in the absence of
     neurological symptoms
     Therapeutic management –
          enzyme replacement
          correction of the anaemia
          consider splenectomy
          bisphosphonates   3

Comment
The sphingolipidoses are a group of disorders caused by the defective catabolism of sphingolipid, leading to an accumulation of various intermediatory degradation products. The accumulation of these molecules occurs within the lysosomes of specific tissues, such as the central nervous system, the liver, spleen, lungs, and the bone marrow which, in turn, produces varying patterns of clinical presentation. In the diseases affecting the central nervous

system, there is often retinal involvement, with the characteristic 'cherry red spot' at the macula. Gaucher's disease is due to glucocerebrocidase deficiency, and has three clinical variants, all of which present with hepatosplenomegaly and the pathognomonic Gaucher cells in the bone marrow. The commonest variant does not involve the nervous system and presents in childhood with hepatomegaly, massive splenomegaly and symptoms secondary to splenic enlargement and bone marrow infiltration. Treatment with enzyme replacement, using macrophage targeted glucocerebrocidase, and bisphosphonates, which improve the bony complications, have both improved overall prognosis. Patients with severe marrow dysfunction require bone marrow transplant. The variants that affect the central nervous system present with seizures, cognitive impairment and focal neurological deficit. The more malignant of the two is associated with pulmonary infiltration, leading to recurrent sepsis and death in the first year of life.

Answer 7 **Marks**

(a)   Autosomal recessive   1

(b)   High arched palate, lens dislocation, genu valgum, scoliosis
       Pectus carinatum is a 'pigeon chest'   4

(c)   Presenting complications is a left calf DVT, with associated
       pulmonary embolism
       Therapeutic management –
              IV access
              Anticoagulate – initially with intravenous heparin,
                     then with warfarin (aiming for an INR of 2–3)
              Analgesia   5

Comment
Homocystinuria is an aminoacidopathy arising due to an enzyme deficiency in the methionine/cysteine pathway. The defective gene is on chromosome 21. It usually presents in late childhood or early adulthood, with low IQ, lens dislocation, skeletal abnormalities and thromboembolic disease. Visual problems are common, arising due to the lens dislocation, glaucoma and retinal detachment. The patients share several features of Marfan's syndrome, but are distinguished by their low IQ. Classically they have a thrombotic tendency, and commonly present with DVT and pulmonary emboli. There is also a predisposition to premature atheromatous disease. Treatment is based on reducing the levels of methionine and homocysteine by the use of oral

pyridoxine. In those unresponsive to this treatment, a methionine free, low protein diet is used.

Answer 8   **Marks**

(a)   Metabolic acidosis
        Liver failure
        Circulatory failure
        Renal failure   3

(b)   Correct extracellular fluid and electrolyte deficits via Na^+
                and water depletion by IV isotonic NaCl solution
        Isotonic $NaHCO_3$ solution to replace impaired renal
                regeneration of bicarbonate; this also has a positive
                inotropic effect on the heart
        Dialysis may be required if treatment induces sodium
                overload   4

(c)   Methanol, ethanol
        Ethylene glycol
        Paraldehyde
        Metformin
        Paracetamol   3

Comment
The correction of acidosis by $NaHCO_3$ infusion may improve cardiac function and peripheral circulation, alleviate hyperventilation and correct hyper-kalaemia. However, rapid alkalinisation in an effort to lower H^+ may reduce cerebral blood flow and reduce oxygenation of the blood. $NaHCO_3$ as an alkalinising agent may also cause Na overload and, paradoxically, may acutely increase intracellular acidosis by $\uparrow$ PCO_2. Liver and renal function must be closely monitored.

Answer 9   **Marks**

(a)   Lactic acidosis due to increased production of lactic acid in
                severe exercise leading to lactic acid accumulation
                in tissues, producing a metabolic acidosis
        Dehydration and salt depletion due to loss of water and salt
                in sweat during severe exercise, particularly in hot
                weather   4

(b)   Administer oxygen by face mask to convert lactic acid to
              pyruvic acid and reduce air hunger
       IV infusion of isotonic dextrose saline to maintain circulatory
              volume and to provide substrate for aerobic metabolism
       Provide warmth with blankets to prevent heat loss from
              chilling   2

(c)   Dehydration and Na loss – assessed by serum U&E
              and corrected by appropriate IV fluid therapy
       Metabolic acidosis assessed by ABG would correct itself
              as accumulated lactic acid is progressively oxidized
              to pyruvic acid and increased respiratory effort washes
              out the CO_2 4

Comment
Lactic acidosis occurs in otherwise healthy individuals as a result of shock leading to circulatory failure, or severe exercise resulting in anaerobic metabolism in muscle tissue, both of which result in lactic acid accumulation. The use of $NaHCO_3$ infusion to correct the acidosis is hazardous: although it may improve cardiac output and peripheral circulation and correct hyperkalaemia, it shifts the O_2 dissociation curve to the left and reduces cerebral perfusion, thereby precipitating cerebral hypoxia.

CHAPTER 3: NEUROLOGY ANSWERS

Answer 1   **Marks**

(a)   Right-sided cerebrovascular accident (CVA)
       Right middle cerebral artery   2

(b)   UMN   LMN
       Bulk   Normal   Normal or wasted
       Tone   Increased   Decreased
                       hypertonia   hypotonia
       Reflexes   Hyper-reflexia   Hypo-reflexia
                       +/– clonus
       Plantars   Extensor   Flexor
                       (upgoing)   (downgoing)   2

(c)   Investigations – FBC, U+Es, glucose, ESR, lipid profile
       ECG
       CXR
       CT head scan
       Consider Doppler USS of the carotids +/- angiography
       Therapeutic management will be based on the cause of the
       stroke, which is confirmed by CT scan
       In thromboembolic stroke
                       – add aspirin 300 mg o.d.
                       – consider anticoagulation with warfarin
       All stroke patients require rehabilitation involving
       physiotherapy, occupational therapy, speech therapy, and
       liaison between district services and social workers,
       i.e. the multidisciplinary team.   3

Comment

Cerebrovascular disease remains one of the three primary causes of death in the Western world, with an annual incidence of approximately 2:1000 of the population. A stroke is defined as 'an acute episode of focal or global loss of cerebral function, lasting for more than 24 hours, or as the principal cause of death'. There are three main causes:

- Cerebral infarction – this accounts for 80% of all strokes
- Intracerebral haemorrhage – 10%
- Subarachnoid haemorrhage – 10%

The risk factors for stroke include:

- Hypertension – this is the main aetiological risk factor and its control has a greater effect than in cardiovascular disease

- Increasing age
- Smoking
- Alcohol abuse
- Cardiac disease – ischaemic, valvular disease, paroxysmal tachyarrhythmia, e.g. atrial fibrillation
- Past history of, or known TIAs or CVAs
- Diabetes mellitus
- Hyperlipidaemia
- Peripheral vascular disease
- The oral contraceptive pill – increases risk 2–3-fold
- Hypercoagulable states – hyperosmolar coma
- Malignancy
- Systemic vasculitides – SLE
- Hypotensive episodes – myocardial infarction, during anaesthesia

Answer 2   **Marks**

(a)   Subarachnoid haemorrhage   1

(b)   Migraine
        Stress headache
        Meningitis
        Space occupying lesion
        Sagital sinus thrombosis (particularly if she is on the oral
        contraceptive pill)   3

(c)   Investigations –   FBC, U+Es, glucose
                             CXR
                             CT head scan
                             Consider lumbar puncture
        Therapeutic management –
                             Nurse in a quiet room if possible
                             IV access and fluids
                             Analgesia (opiates if necessary)
                             Nimodipine
                             Neurosurgical opinion   6

Comment
Subarachnoid haemorrhage is responsible for 10% of all strokes. The majority of patients bleed after rupture of a saccular intracranial aneurysm or from an arteriovenous malformation. Clinically the patient presents with a severe

headache, which starts abruptly and is often described as the worst headache they have ever experienced. It may be associated with neck stiffness, meningism and occasionally seizures. Consciousness may be impaired, and the patient may present in coma with larger bleeds. Diagnosis is usually confirmed with CT head scan, which will show blood in the ventricles and subarachnoid space. (Blood appears as a white collection on an unenhanced scan.) A lumbar puncture may be required if the scan is unhelpful and, if confirmatory, will show blood in all three CSF samples. A sample taken 24 hours or more after the initial symptoms may appear yellow in colour, termed xanthochromia. Fifty per cent of patients will die within one month of their initial episode. Neurosurgical intervention should always be considered when the patient is neurologically intact and consciousness is spared. Radiological embolization of arteriovenous malformations now offers a less invasive method of treatment. The calcium channel blocker, nimodipine, is recommended for secondary prophylaxis, as it stops vasospasm causing secondary bleeds. It may be given orally or intravenously depending on the patient's level of consciousness.

Answer 3   **Marks**

(a)   Horner's syndrome
       Loss of the sympathetic nerve supply to the eye   2

(b) (i) An apical malignant tumour in the right lung
         (Pancoast's tumour)   1
    (ii) Brainstem CVA
         Syringomyelia
         Accidental or surgical trauma to the neck   3

(c)   A right IIIrd nerve palsy causes the full ptosis, with the
       action of the unopposed superior oblique and lateral rectus
       muscles causing the eye to turn down and out
       Loss of the parasympathetic nerve supply causes the fixed,
       dilated pupil
       Causes –   Diabetes mellitus
                   Mononeuritis multiplex
                   CVA   4

Comment
The Horner's syndrome consists of enophthalmos, the globe of the eye is sunken in the orbit, pupillary constriction, partial ptosis and anhydrosis, or loss of sweating on the affected side of the face (this is dependent on whether

the interruption of the nerve supply is above or below the cervical sympathetic ganglion). The syndrome arises due to an interruption in the sympathetic nerve supply to the eye. This may arise anywhere along its course from the midbrain, down through the brainstem and cervical cord, as it emerges from the spine at T1, and then as it passes up through the neck. Common lesions are:

- **Brain stem** – CVA, tumours, syringobulbia
- **Cervical cord** – tumour, syringomyelia
- **T1 lesion** – Pancoast's tumour, benign apical lung disease, e.g. TB or abscess
- **In the neck** – operative or accidental cervical trauma.

In apical lung disease, the brachial plexus may also be involved leading to pain, parasthesiae and loss of sensation along the ulnar border of the forearm and the medial (ulnar) two fingers, as well as wasting of the intrinsic muscles of the hand. Third nerve palsies may occur in isolation or with loss of the accompanying parasympathetic nerve supply. If the parasympathetic supply is unaffected this is termed 'pupillary sparing', which arises principally due to a vascular event.

Answer 4   **Marks**

(a) (i) Left facial (VIIth) nerve palsy   1
    (ii) Lower motor neurone lesions cause a total hemifacial palsy,
       whereas upper motor neurone lesions have sparing of the
       forehead and the upper eyelid   2

(b)   Idiopathic
      Parotid infiltration
      Pontine tumours and CVAs
      Mononeuritis multiplex   4

(c)   Bell's palsy
      In early presentations high dose steroids are advocated
      Most will resolve spontaneously   3

Comment

Facial nerve palsy is a common cranial nerve lesion, most often presenting as part of a cerebrovascular event. The nerve innervates the muscles of facial expression, and supplies taste sensation to the anterior two-thirds of the tongue. The facial nucleus lies within the pons and receives bilateral motor cortex supply. Thus lesions which are supranuclear cause an upper motor neurone palsy and have sparing of the superior aspects of the face due to contralateral nerve supply. Common causes of a facial palsy are:

- Upper motor neurone – Pontine CVA, tumours, Cerebral cortex and internal capsule CVAs
- Lower motor neurone – Idiopathic (Bell's palsy), Cerebellopontine angle tumours, Ramsey–Hunt syndrome (this is caused by a herpes zoster infection), Basal skull fracture, Parotid infiltration (e.g. sarcoid, lymphoma, amyloid), Iatrogenic injury during facial and parotid surgery, Mononeuritis multiplex (e.g. diabetes mellitus, systemic vasculitides)

Answer 5	**Marks**
(a) (i) Peripheral sensory neuropathy	1
(ii) Malignancy	
Alcohol abuse	2
(b) Light touch, proprioception and vibration – dorsal columns	
Pinprick (pain) and temperature – spinothalamic tract	3
(c) Stroke (CVA)	
Mononeuritis multiplex	
Autonomic neuropathy	
Cranial nerve palsies	
Argyll Robertson pupil	4

Comment

Peripheral neuropathy is a common sequelae of poorly controlled diabetes mellitus. It was previously thought to be due to microvascular disease, but more recent work has concluded that it is probably due to abnormal axonal metabolism of carbohydrate, which causes secondary damage to the nerve conduction. Common causes of neuropathy are:

- Sensory neuropathy – Idiopathic – 50% of cases; Metabolic – B12 deficiency, uraemia, diabetes mellitus; Drugs – isoniazid, phenytoin, chloramphenicol; Alcohol associated – thiamine (vitamin B1) deficiency; Malignancy – as part of a paraneoplastic phenomenon
- Motor neuropathy – Heavy metal toxicity – lead, mercury; Drugs – gold, amphoterecin; Motor neurone disease; Malignancy – paraneoplastic phenomenon, Guillain–Barré syndrome

Answer 6   **Marks**

(a)   Benign and malignant tumours
        Obstructing hydrocephalus
        Benign intracranial hypertension   3

(b)   CT or MRI scan of the brain (with contrast)
        CXR
        FBC with blood film and differential
        If appropriate – HIV test with pre-test counselling   3

(c)   Neurosurgery –   drainage of abscess
                              biopsy of mass
                              excision of accessible masses
        Radiotherapy – curative, palliative or adjuvant
        Chemotherapy – monotherapy or adjuvant
        Medical – antibiotics for abscesses   4

Comment

This woman gives a history suggestive of raised intracranial pressure with headache, nausea and vomiting, visual disturbance and seizures which are common presenting symptoms. Focal neurological deficit may present as third and sixth cranial nerve palsies with an ipsilateral hemiparesis, and are known as 'false localizing signs'. They are due to increasing intracranial pressure stretching the nerves at the base of the skull. Causes of raised intracranial pressure include

- Infection (meningitis, abscess), Benign tumours (meningioma, neurofibroma), Malignant tumours (primary – astrocytoma, glioma, neuroblastoma, lymphoma; secondary – cervical, breast, lung)

Obstructing hydrocephalus may be secondary to:

- Tumours of the posterior fossa
- Subarachnoid haemorrhage
- Tuberculous meningitis
- Colloid cyst of the third ventricle

Benign intracranial hypertension is an idiopathic disorder, commonly seen in young women. It is thought to be related to obesity and the oral contraceptive pill. Patients present with severe headaches for which the only abnormality found is raised intracranial pressure. Treatment is based on stopping the pill, weight reduction and diuretics. Normal pressure hydrocephalus is a syndrome seen principally in the elderly, which presents with a classical triad of worsening confusion, urinary incontinence and dyspraxia. The diagnosis is confirmed by CT head scan which shows dilatation of the ventricles without evidence of cerebral atrophy. Lumbar puncture will confirm normal manometry. Although single manometry readings are normal, these patients often have periods of raised intracranial pressure and may benefit from insertion of a ventriculoperitoneal shunt.

Answer 7   **Marks**

(a)   Epilepsy – probably absence seizure   1

(b)   FBC, U+Es, glucose, calcium and magnesium
        CXR
        CT head scan
        EEG
        Lumbar puncture   5

(c)   Sodium valproate – ataxia, jaundice
        Carbamazepine – gynaecomastia, GI upset
        Phenytoin – seizures, peripheral neuropathy, gingival,
                hyperplasia, folate deficiency
        Phenobarbitone – megaloblastic anaemia, confusion, sedation
        Lamotrigine – rashes, fever
        Vigabatrin – drowsiness, confusion
        Gabapentin – drowsiness, ataxia   4

Comment
Epilepsy is a common neurological disorder, with an annual incidence of 80:100,000 cases in the UK. It is defined as two or more non-febrile seizures. Epilepsy is classified into three groups, which are subdivided by the characteristics of the seizures:
•   **Partial seizures** are caused by the activation of a localized, definable group of neurones, sited within one cerebral hemisphere. They are subdivided into **Simple partial seizures** – these are characterized by the site of the abnormal activity, e.g. pure motor, sensory or psychic phenomena. They are not associated with loss of consciousness; **Complex partial seizures** – these have the symptoms of simple seizures, but are associated with an impairment of consciousness; **Secondary generalized seizures** – these begin with features of simple or complex seizures, which then become generalized with tonic–clonic episodes. The initial partial element may be so shortlived that it may be only evident on the EEG.

- **Generalized seizures** arise due to symmetrical abnormal neuronal activation in the cerebral hemispheres. They are subdivided into **Absence seizures** – these are subdivided into typical and atypical. Typical absence seizures are characterized by their EEG discharge of 3Hz 'spike and waves', and were formerly known as *petit mal* seizures. Both are associated with impaired consciousness, with typical seizures often associated with complex patterns of movement and behaviour; **Myoclonic seizures** – these are subdivided into tonic–clonic (formerly known as *grand mal* seizures), tonic and clonic seizures. They are associated with impairment of consciousness.

Classically tonic–clonic seizures are associated with biting of the tongue and incontinence of urine.

Answer 8   **Marks**

(a)   Motor neurone disease
       Progressive bulbar palsy   3

(b)   EMG
       Myelogram
       Muscle biopsy
       MRI of the cervical spine and brainstem
       Lumbar puncture   3

(c)   Once other diagnoses have been excluded:
       An experienced physician should discuss the prognosis, and
             counsel the patient and family
       Speech therapist to improve articulation and swallowing
       Physiotherapy and occupational therapy
       Nutrition support and dietary advice, may require gastrostomy
             feeding
       Computer-assisted communication for speech failure or severe
             dysarthria
       Terminal care – community support, e.g. Macmillan nurses,
             hospice care   4

Comment

Motor neurone disease is an idiopathic, progressive neurological disorder, characterized by a mixture of upper and lower motor neurone signs. There are never associated sensory or cerebellar signs and the ocular movements are preserved. It is a diagnosis of exclusion as there are no definitive tests for the disorder and the diagnosis can therefore only be inferred clinically and by negative investigations for the main differential diagnoses. MRI of the cervical spine and brainstem, with or without myelography, is the principal investigation, as this will exclude the main differential, cervical spondylosis with associated radiculomyelopathy. Motor neurone disease is one of the main causes of a progressive bulbar palsy, i.e. palsies of the IXth to XIIth cranial nerves which lie within the medulla or bulb of the brainstem. Patients present with 'nasal' speech and dysarthria, and dysphagia to both solids and liquids. The tongue is wasted and flaccid and there is weakness of palatal movement. Other causes include syringobulbia, Guillain–Barré syndrome and poliomyelitis. Motor neurone disease carries a poor prognosis and there remains no specific treatment, but NICE (National Institute for Clinical Excellence) have recently approved the use of Riluzole [Rilutek] which has been shown to slow the progression of the disease. Palliation is the main aim of therapy, requiring a multidisciplinary approach. The prognosis is mainly dependent on the involvement of the bulbar muscles. In cases where the initial symptoms are spinal, 15% survive to 5 years; if there are associated bulbar symptoms this falls to approximately 5%.

Answer 9 **Marks**

(a) Myasthenia gravis
     Autoimmune disease – autoantibodies(IgG), directed against
     the postsynaptic acetylcholine (ACh) receptor   3

(b) Tensilon (edrophonium) test
     Auto antibody screen including the IgG directed against the
     ACh receptor   2

(c) Oral anticholinesterases, e.g. pyridostigmine
     Immunosuppresents – steroids and azothioprine
     Thymectomy – in patients under 40 years old
     Plasma exchange – in short term control
     Atropine – cholinergic crisis   5

Comment
Myasthenia gravis is an autoimmune disease caused by an autoantibody IgG, directed against the postsynaptic acetylcholine receptor. It is associated with several other autoimmune disorders including thyrotoxicosis and myxoedema, pernicious anaemia, rheumatoid arthritis and SLE. It occurs at most ages, but has a peak incidence at 30. As with most autoimmune disorders it is

more common in women. The thymus gland is often abnormal in these patients, especially in those under 40 years old. 60–70% have thymic hyperplasia and 10% develop a thymoma. This group of patients commonly has an additional autoantibody directed against striated muscle. A thymectomy is recommended in this group, especially in the under 40s. The diagnosis is usually confirmed by a Tensilon test. An intravenous injection of an anticholinesterase (edrophonium) is given, which produces an instant improvement. If the initial injection fails to do so, a further larger bolus can be given. Lambert–Eaton syndrome is a malignant associated myasthenic syndrome, most often occurring as a result of a small cell tumour of the lung. Unlike the primary disorder, the IgG is directed against the presynaptic calcium channels, and so it does not respond to anticholinesterases. Treatment is directed at the underlying tumour and increasing the action potential duration and the amount of neurotransmitter released using the drug 3,4 diaminopyridine.

Answer 10   **Marks**

(a)   Parkinson's disease   2
       Dopamine

(b)   Arteriosclerotic Parkinson syndrome
       Drug induced parkinsonism
       Progressive supranuclear palsy (Steele–Richardson–Olszewski
       syndrome)   2

(c)   L-dopa – nausea, confusion, postural hypotension
       Selegeline – confusion, hypotension
       Pergolide – hallucination
       Apomorphine – hallucination, nausea
       Bromocriptine – confusion   6

Comment
Parkinson's disease is a common neurological disorder, particularly in the elderly, where its prevalence is 1:200. It classically presents with an insidious onset of bradykinesia, rigidity and tremor, associated with postural and gait problems. This combination leads to increasing difficulties with mobility and falls. Pathologically it is characterized by an idiopathic loss of dopaminergic cells within the substantia nigra, and the presence of eosinophilic inclusions, known as Lewy bodies. In Parkinsonism, the extra-pyramidal, akinetic-rigidity symptoms arise in relation to other diffuse brain disease, such as

multi-infarct dementia, Alzheimer's disease, Lewy body dementia, and Creutzfeld–Jakob disease. Parkinsonism may also arise secondary to various toxic insults to the brain, e.g. anoxia, carbon monoxide poisoning and drugs, such as antipsychotics and anti-emetics. Parkinson's disease is treated initially with a combination of l-dopa and a peripheral dopa decarboxylase inhibitor, which will improve symptoms, but do not influence the progression of the disease. As the disorder progresses, other agents may be employed. These include the dopamine agonists pergolide, lisuride and bromocriptine, and the MAOI type B, selegeline. In difficult cases, where there is a poor response to medication, or in advanced disease, a continuous subcutaneous infusion of apomorphine may be used. Surgical intervention may also be tried in these cases, using stereotaxic thalamotomy and thalamic stimulation. The implantation of foetal dopaminergic tissue remains controversial.

Answer 11	**Marks**
(a) (i) X-linked recessive	1
(ii) Becker's muscular dystrophy Lesch–Nyhan syndrome Haemophilia A Red–green colour blindness	2
(b) CPK Muscle biopsy EMG	3
(c) Drugs, e.g. steroids Infection – poliomyelitis Endocrine – Cushing's syndrome, hypothyroidism Toxins – alcohol	4

Comment

Duchenne's muscular dystrophy is classically an X-linked recessive disorder, although one-third of cases arise due to spontaneous mutation. The responsible gene defect is located in the Xp21 region of the X chromosome. The condition presents in early childhood with wasting of the proximal limb musculature, and associated weakness. The child walks with a 'waddling' gait and classically cannot 'walk' their hands up their legs to a standing position (Gower's sign). The proximal wasting is often associated with enlargement of the calves, termed pseudohypertrophy. The disorder is progressive and the child is often confined to a wheelchair by the age of 10, with death occurring by the age of 20 due to cardiac and respiratory muscle involvement. Becker's muscular dystrophy is a more benign disorder, which presents usually in the second to third decade of life and progresses slowly with the patient usually confined to a wheelchair by the age of 40–50.

Answer 12   **Marks**

(a)   Multiple sclerosis
        Plaques of demyelination within the central nervous system   2

(b)   CSF for oligoclonal bands
        MRI of the cervical spine and brainstem to demonstrate
                plaques of demyelination
        Visual evoked responses (VER) show delayed conduction
                between the retina and the occipital cortex   3

(c)   Education about the disease and prognosis for patient and
                family
        In relapses – high dose IV methylprednisolone
        Symptom relief and help for:
                incontinence
                spasticity
                immobility
                sexual dysfunction
        Social support for patient and family   5

Comment

Multiple sclerosis is an idiopathic disorder, causing demyelination within the central nervous system. It presents between the ages of 20–40 years. It is a disease principally of northern Europeans, and the immigrant populations of South Africa and Australasia that descended from them. The disease is thought to be due to an abnormal immune response to environmental agents, such as viruses, as a direct result or as a consequence of abnormal gene sequencing. Viral agents implicated in this immune reaction include measles, mumps, rubella and EBV. The disease is divided clinically into a chronic progressive disorder and a rapid relapsing/remitting one. Prognosis is at present uninfluenced by any treatments, and therapy is principally aimed at palliation of the complications and delay of relapses with immuno-suppressants. Relapses are shortened in duration by high dose intravenous steroids. Beta interferon is the most promising of the conventional therapies, and work is also continuing into the use of monoclonal antibody therapy directed against the abnormal immunological responses.

Answer 13   **Marks**

(a) (i) This woman has spinal metastases from her colonic
     carcinoma   1

  (ii) Extrinsic and intrinsic spinal cord lesions
     Demyelination
     Trauma   2

(b) T10 is approximately the level of the umbilicus
    X-rays of the thoracic and lumbar spine
    Radioisotope bone scan
    MRI +/– myelography of the spinal cord   4

(c) Management –   Neurosurgical decompression of the cord
                  Local radiotherapy to bony metastases
                  Palliation of symptoms –
                        urinary catheter for incontinence
                        laxatives for constipation
                        analgesia
                  Multidisciplinary palliative care team   3

Comment

A spastic paraparesis may present insidiously, worsening over several months, or as an acute event. In all cases it is essential to define whether a sensory level is present, and to what extent bladder and anal sphincter control are affected. Common causes of a spastic paraparesis are:

- Extrinsic cord compression – this is principally due to infiltration or collapse of the vertebral bodies. Common causes include: Metastases, e.g. bronchus, breast, prostate, thyroid and colon, Myeloma, Paget's disease of the bone, Pott's disease of the spine (tuberculosis), Spondylolysthesis
- Other causes of external compression are tumours, e.g. neurofibroma, meningioma and abscesses
- Intrinsic cord lesions (Tumours, e.g. ependymoma, glioma, teratoma, Demyelination, Syringomyelia, Metabolic, e.g. B12 deficiency, Vascular, e.g. anterior spinal artery occlusion)

Answer 14   **Marks**

(a) (i) Guillain–Barré syndrome   1
   (ii) Paraneoplastic syndrome
      Infective, e.g. HIV
      Hereditary sensorimotor neuropathy   2

(b)   Hypotonia with loss of power
     Diminished or absent patella and ankle reflexes
     Flexor plantar responses
     Fasciculation may occur   3

(c)   Management –
     Usually supportive treatment only, i.e. nutrition, fluids, bed rest
     Treat any reversible cause, e.g. *Mycoplasma pneumoniae*
     Monitor respiratory function with regular spirometry
     May require assisted ventilation
     If prolonged will require nutritional support
     If severe, consider plasma exchange and IV human
          immunoglobulin   4

Comment

Guillain–Barré syndrome is a post-infective polyneuropathy, which has recently been closely linked to *Campylobacter jejuni* and HIV infection, particularly in its more malignant form. Other implicated organisms include EBV, CMV, enterovirus and *Mycoplasma pneumoniae*. In 40% of cases there is no identifiable preceding cause. The disorder commonly presents 1–3 weeks after the onset of the infection, with distal motor and sensory symptoms and signs. In 20% of cases the symptoms ascend to involve the respiratory and facial muscles, causing acute respiratory failure and the need for assisted ventilation. In these severe cases plasma exchange and human immunoglobulin are often required. High dose steroids are commonly given but do not influence the outcome. Other causes of a sensorimotor neuropathy include:

*   Hereditary sensorimotor neuropathies (e.g. Charcot–Marie–Tooth disease)
*   Malignancy (paraneoplastic syndrome)
*   Infection (HIV, Lyme's disease, diphtheria)
*   Amyloid

Answer 15   **Marks**

(a)   Autosomal dominant
        1:2 chance   2

(b)   Chorea – continuous, irregular movements which may be
        explosive in nature, and flit from one part of the body to
        another
        Other causes –   Sydenham's chorea
                                      Chorea gravidarum
                                      Drugs, e.g. neuroleptics
                                      Thyrotoxicosis   4

(c)   Genetic counselling and screening of patient and family
        Exclude any treatable causes
        Palliation of symptoms – phenothiazines and tetrabenazine
                are given for the chorea; antipsychotics
        Social support for family and patient
        Consider nursing home care if family are unable to cope with
                patient at home   4

Comment

Huntington's chorea is a progressive neurological disorder, characterized by a relentlessly progressive dementia and choreiform movements. There are adult and childhood forms, the early onset being between 10–20 and the adult form between 30–50 years. The abnormal gene locus has been isolated to the short arm of chromosome 4, which has allowed genetic screening of family members, including the foetus *in utero*. Pathologically the disorder is characterized by loss of GABA and ACh within the corpus striatum and ACE and metenkephalin within the substantia nigra. The loss of these neurotransmitters leads to a relative excess of dopaminergic activity which is thought to be responsible for the choreiform movements. Other causes of chorea include:

- Sydenham's chorea (this is associated with rheumatic fever but may occur in association with other disorders. Chorea gravidarum is regarded as a variant of this condition and occurs in pregnancy and with users of the oral contraceptive pill)
- Drugs (neuroleptics, anticonvulsants)
- Toxins (alcohol)
- Benign hereditary chorea
- Endocrine disorders (thyrotoxicosis, hypoparathyroidism)

- Metabolic (hypernatraemia)
- Intra-cranial haemorrhage and thromboembolic strokes
- Polycythaemia rubra vera

Answer 16   **Marks**

(a)   Ataxic, widebased gait
        Past pointing
        Intention tremor
        Dysdiadochokinesis
        Cerebellar (staccato) speech
        Horizontal nystagmus   2

(b)   Chronic alcohol abuse
        Phenytoin toxicity   2

(c)   Investigations –   FBC with MCV
                                        LFTs including gamma GT
                                        Phenytoin level
        Medications –
                                        Diazepam or chlormethiazole for withdrawal symptoms
                                        Multivitamins and thiamine   6

Comment

Cerebellar lesions may present with ipsilateral or bilateral signs, depending on the cause. They are characterized by problems of movement control and co-ordination. Dysmetria is the inability to control the force, direction and distance of a movement, whilst dysdiadochokinesia is the inability to perform rapid alternating movements. Patients with cerebellar lesions classically have staccato speech and coarse, horizontal nystagmus; they may also have hypotonia and diminished reflexes. Common causes of cerebellar lesions include:

- Cerebellar infarction or haemorrhage
- Cerebellar abscess
- Demyelination
- Toxins (e.g. alcohol, lead, carbon monoxide)
- Drugs (e.g. anticonvulsants)
- Inherited disorders (e.g. Friedreich's ataxia, ataxia telangiectasia)
- Anatomical abnormalities (e.g. Arnold–Chiari malformation, Dandy Walker syndrome)
- Malignancy (primary and secondary tumours; a paraneoplastic syndrome)

CHAPTER 4: ENDOCRINOLOGY ANSWERS

Answer 1   **Marks**

(a) (i)   Primary hypothyroidism   1
     (ii) Atrophic or autoimmune thyroiditis
           Hashimoto's thyroiditis
           Iodine deficiency
           Dyshormonogenesis   2

(b) Replacement therapy with oral thyroxine for life, with a
     starting dose of 0.025–0.05 mg/day. The aim of therapy is
     to restore TSH to within normal levels by slowly increasing
     the dose over several months   3

(c) Myxoedematous coma is a medical emergency. Admit,
     reverse hypothermia, monitor cardiac and respiratory function.
     Administer tri-iodothyronine IV 0.025 mg as a bolus,
     followed by 0.025 mg 8-hourly until there is sustained
     clinical improvement before substituting with oral thyroxine   4

Comment
Autoimmune hypothyroidism is the commonest cause of glandular under-
activity and is due to microsomal autoantibodies destroying the gland, with
eventual atrophy and fibrosis. In Hashimoto's disease the autoantibodies are
associated with glandular destruction and regeneration, leading to goitre
formation. The mortality in severe hypothyroidism in the elderly is significant
and may manifest as confusion dementia or coma. Hypothermia, cardiac
failure, hypoventilation, hypocalcaemia and hyponatraemia may all be
present, and the patient should be managed in an intensive therapy unit.

Answer 2   **Marks**

(a) Graves' disease. Here, hyperthyroidism results from the
     production of IgG microsomal antibodies against TSH
     receptors on the thyroid follicular cell, which stimulates
     thyroid hormone production and goitre formation. Long-acting
     thyroid stimulating anti-bodies are also found in the serum of
     patients but their role is uncertain   3

(b) Goitre (diffuse or nodular) ± bruit/thrill
     Sinus tachycardia, atrial fibrillation
     Proximal myopathy, hyperreflexia

Lid lag and retraction
Exophthalmus, ophthalmoplegia
Papilloedema, loss of visual acuity, diplopia
Amenorrhoea (infertility)
Pretibial myxoedema
Hands: tremor, sweating, increased pulse pressure, onychyolysis,
    thyroid acropachy   3

(c)

Treatment	Complications
Anti-thyroid agents, viz carbimazole	Hypersensitivity, agranulocytosis > 50% relapse within two years of stopping therapy
Subtotal thryoidectomy	Hypoparathyroidism Hypothyroidism Recurrent laryngeal nerve injury
Radioiodine therapy	Hypothyroidism: 40% incidence in 1st year, 80% incidence after 15 years Not given to women of child-bearing age 4

Comment

Graves' disease is an autoimmune disease of the thyroid. The patient may be biochemically and clinically hyper-, hypo- or euthyroid. It is associated with other autoimmune disorders, and is characterized by the triad of eye signs (Graves' orbitopathy) pretibial myxoedema and thyroid acropachy. The natural history of the disease is one of fluctuation, with relapses and remissions. Subtotal thyroidectomy is the treatment of choice for the hyperactive gland. Preoperative management is aimed at achieving a euthyroid state and to reduce glandular vascularity and to avoid peri-operative complications. Eye signs, however, may not be reversed by thyroidectomy and may require peri-orbital decompression. When surgery is not desired or is contraindicated the patient is started on carbimazole or propylthiouracil, and this is continued for 12–18 months. In younger patients therapy is then stopped; relapse may occur immediately or, on occasion, after many years. In older patients (> 40 years of age) or in those women who have completed their families, radioactive iodine therapy is given. This may require admission but can be given as an outpatient.

Answer 3   **Marks**

(a)   (i)   Prolactin secreting tumour of the pituitary   1
       (ii)   Pregnancy
              Lactation   2

(b)   Metaclopramide
       Oestrogens
       Dopamine antagonists
       Phenothiazines, e.g. chlorpromazine
       Butyrophenones, e.g. haloperidol
       Dopamine depleting agents
       Reserpine, methyldopa   3

(c)   Medical: Dopamine agonist therapy with bromocriptine
       (dose: 2.5 mg p.o. tid with meals); start with a low dose of
       1.25 mg daily, with gradual increments; may be given as a
       pessary if poorly tolerated
       Surgical: Transphenoidal removal of selected tumours, viz
       cystic macroadenomas
       Radiotherapy: By external beam radiation or transphenoidal
       implantation of radioactive yttrium needles   4

Comment

Prolactin secretion differs from other anterior pituitary hormones in that it is
under predominantly dopaminergic inhibitory control by the hypothalamus.
Bromocriptine therapy therefore effectively lowers prolactin levels and
shrinks large tumours, which may subsequently be treated by transphenoidal
surgery or radiotherapy. Serum prolactin levels must be checked in cases of
unexplained amenorrhoea or irregular periods associated with infertility or, in
men, gynaecomastia with headaches or visual impairment.

Answer 4   **Marks**

(a)   (i)   Acromegaly; acidophil or acidophil and chromophobe
              mixed adenoma of the anterior pituitary   2
       (ii)   Baseline serum, prolactin and glucose levels followed
              by an oral glucose tolerance test which would show a
              paradoxical rise in growth hormone level along with
              the rise in blood glucose   2

(b)   Coarsened facial features – broadened nose, lips and tongue
        Visceromegaly (e.g. thyroid, heart, liver, spleen)
        Frontal bossing, increased interdental separation, overbiting,
            enlarged mandible
        Hypertension
        Diabetes mellitus
        Kyphosis, arthropathy, proximal myopathy
        Carpal tunnel syndrome   3

(c)   Medical: Initial treatment with Octreotide (somatostatin
        analogue) SC or bromocriptine PO
        Surgical: Transphenoidal removal of adenoma
        Radiotherapy: External beam or yttrium implants stops
        tumour growth and lowers growth hormone levels   3

Comment
Gigantism and acromegaly are the clinical states produced by growth
hormone hypersecretion before and after the fusion of epiphyseal cartilages.
Tumour expansion produces headaches and in 30% of all patients the tumour
affects adjacent pituitary function, viz compression of the anterior pituitary
causes hypothyroidism, hypogonadism and Addison's disease. Local
complications are due to suprasellar extension of the tumour, and
compression of the optic chiasma may cause several visual field defects,
including bitemporal hemianopia. Cavernous sinus extension may cause III,
IV, V and VI nerve compression and palsy. Extension to the pituitary stalk
may stop the dopaminergic inhibition of prolactin from the hypothalamus,
leading to hyperprolactinaemia.

Answer 5   **Marks**

(a)   Cushing's syndrome is defined as the symptoms and signs
        associated with prolonged inappropriate elevation of free
        plasma corticosteroid levels   2

(b)   Muscle weakness: Gluconeogenesis leads to loss of muscle
        protein and proximal myopathy
        Skin bruising: Collagen breakdown due to glucocorticoid
        excess leads to thinning of the skin and fragility of skin blood
        vessels
        Hypertension: Glucocorticoid excess increases plasma volume
        and enhances vascular responsiveness to noradrenalin

Impaired glucose tolerance: due to increased gluco-neogenesis
produced by excess glucocorticoids   4

(c)   Plasma ACTH level at 0900 hrs:
        Normal range (10–80 ng/l) suggests a pituitary source
        Moderate elevation (80–300 ng/l) indicates an extra-pituitary
        source (viz adrenals) and high levels (>300 ng/l) are due to
        ectopic ACTH syndrome (viz bronchial carcinoma)
        Low versus high dose dexamethasone suppression test:
        low dose enzyme inhibitor metyrapone blocks cortisol biosynthesis
        and markedly elevates plasma ACTH, whereas high dose
        dexamethasone suppression test lowers plasma ACTH in
        pituitary dependent states   4

Comment
Cushing's syndrome may be ACTH-dependent, such as in pituitary-dependent
adrenal hyperplasia, or ACTH-independent, as in functional adrenal tumours
and ectopic ACTH syndrome. Dexamethasone suppresses ACTH production
by a negative feedback of corticosteroids on the hypothalamus and pituitary.
A reduction of ACTH output is assessed by the fall in these corticosteroids.
The low dose test may be used to differentiate Cushing's syndrome from
normality, whereas the high dose test usually distinguishes the different
causes (e.g. ectopic or adrenal disease). Cushing's syndrome due to pituitary
or adrenal lesions is four times more common in women. Untreated,
Cushing's syndrome has a 50% five-year fatality rate.

Answer 6   **Marks**

(a)   Primary: Addison's disease
        Enzyme defects
        Secondary: hypothalamic/pituitary disease
        Glucocorticoid therapy   3

(b)   Fever, vitiligo
        Nausea, anorexia, postural hypotension, vomiting,
        abdominal pain diarrhoea/constipation, depression,
        confusion, myalgia, joint/back pain,
        impotence/amenorrhoea   3

(c)   An 0900 hr plasma ACTH level that is high (>80 ng/l)
        with a low/normal cortisol level confirms primary hypoadrenalism

ACTH stimulation test (short):
> A modified ACTH (tetracosactrin or synacthen) 0.25 mg is given IM. After 30 min in normal subjects the plasma cortisol would exceed 600 nmol/l. A peak of >600 nmol/l or a rise of >330 nmol/l indicates adrenocortical insufficiency and confirms diagnosis   4

Comment

Primary adrenocortical insufficiency is due to destruction of, or damage to, the adrenal glands caused by autoimmune adrenalitis or TB. Secondary insufficiency is due to hypothalamic or pituitary disease resulting in impaired ACTH secretion and subsequent adrenocortical atrophy. An important difference is that in the former, mineralocorticoid production is usually impaired because of destruction of adrenal tissue; in the latter, the zona glomerulosa functions normally and is controlled by the renin-angiotensin pathway. Autoimmune disease is the predominant cause of Addison's disease today and may be associated with other autoimmune diseases affecting the thyroid (Hashimoto's disease, idiopathic myxoedema, autoimmune thyroiditis and Graves' disease), stomach (pernicious anaemia and atrophic gastritis), pancreas (insulin-dependent diabetes), testis and ovary (primary testicular and ovarian failure). Addison's disease is treated with oral hydrocortisone (cortisol) and/or cortisone acetate in daily divided doses, along with fludrocortisone to replace aldosterone. Adrenal crisis requires emergency treatment with IV fluids and IV hydrocortisone. A precipitating cause is usually a superimposed infection requiring active treatment. Patients with Addison's disease must carry a card stating their diagnosis, their GP and the steroid dosage they are on with hospital details and reference number. Some of this information may be worn on a bracelet.

Answer 7   **Marks**

(a)   Excess aldosterone production is due to adrenal adenomas, (Conn's syndrome) or bilateral hyperplasia of the zona glomerulosa and leads to potassium loss and hypertension   3

(b)   Hypokalaemia
Raised plasma aldosterone
Metabolic alkalosis   2

(c)   An adenoma should be surgically removed
Hyperplasia is treated with aldosterone antagonists

spironolactone (100–400 mg/day) or amiloride (10–40 mg/day)
Salt and water depletion require IV saline infusion 3

(d) The renin-angiotensin axis is stimulated by
    (i)   physiological factors such as pregnancy (due to
          progesterone effect) or extra-vascular fluid or salt loss
    (ii)   pathological causes such as nephrotic syndrome,
          cirrhosis with ascites and congestive cardiac failure
          (all lead to a decreased renal perfusion and
          increased renin release) 2

Comment

The syndrome of aldosterone excess may be either primary, due to disease of
the adrenal gland, or secondary, when caused by excessive stimulation of the
adrenal gland by extrinsic disease. The hypertension is caused by sodium
retention and potassium excretion by the kidney under the direct action of
aldosterone. This results in increased plasma and extracellular volumes and
hence increased blood pressure with consequent suppression of plasma renin.
Angiotensin converting enzyme (ACE) inhibitors (captopril, enalapril, etc)
inhibit the conversion of angiotensin I to angiotensin II. The latter stimulates
sympathetic vasoconstriction and aldosterone secretion. Hyperaldosteronism
is a rare cause of hypertension, and on investigating for this disease in these
patients, anti-hypertensive therapy must be stopped for two weeks before-
hand, due to their effects on renin secretion (thiazide diuretics stimulate,
whereas beta-adrenergic receptor blockers inhibit).

Answer 8   **Marks**

(a) Changes in plasma osmolality are sensed by osmoreceptors
     in the anterior hypothalamus. ADH secretion is suppressed
     at levels below 280 m/osmol/Kg producing a water diuresis;
     at 295 m/osmol/Kg maximum antidiuresis is achieved and
     thirst experienced at higher levels 3

(b) Diabetes insipidus is caused by pituitary/hypothalamic
     lesions causing deficient ADH production or by renal
     lesions resulting in the renal tubules becoming unresponsive
     to ADH; the disease is characterized by the passage of large
     amounts of dilute urine and by the presence of constant thirst 3

(c) For pituitary/hypothalamic lesions a vasopressin analogue

(desmopressin) is administered intranasally (10–40 μg) by
titrating the daily dose required to keep the patient in fluid
balance   4

Comment
In cranial diabetes insipidus the cause is either a primary or secondary tumour
in the posterior pituitary and/or hypothalamus. Suprasellar tumours (cranio-
pharyngioma) and metastatic carcinoma (viz breast and lung) may also
produce vasopressin insufficiency. In nephrogenic diabetes insipidus the renal
tubules fail to respond to vasopressin due to a genetic defect (inborn error of
metabolism). Potassium depletion, hypercalcaemia and amyloidosis may also
cause polyuria unresponsive to vasopressin. Lithium therapy for manic
depressive illness may also cause reversible nephrogenic diabetes insipidus.
Syndromes of inappropriate anti-diuretic hormone secretion present as confusion, irritability and, later, fits and coma. The plasma osmolarity is low, with
an abnormally high urine osmolarity. The causes include cranial (head injury,
meningitis, encephalitis), pulmonary (infections and tumours), metabolic
(porphyria, alcohol withdrawal), pancreatic, prostatic and thymic tumours and
drugs (chlorpropamide, vincristine). Symptomatic measures include fluid
restriction to 500–1000 ml/day and drugs to produce a diuresis (e.g.
dimethylchlortetracycline or frusemide).

Answer 9   **Marks**

(a)   Acute hypercalcaemia or hypercalcaemia crisis   2

(b)   Sarcoidosis
       Addison's disease
       Bone diseases – multiple myeloma, osteoclastoma,
       osteitis fibrosa
       Malignancies of the breast, kidney, lung, thyroid, ovary
       and colon   3

(c)   Rehydrate with 4–6 l of normal saline in the first 24 hours,
       with correction of any associated deficiencies; fluid therapy
       alone would lower Ca^{2+} levels to 3.0 mmol/l within 72 hours;
       IV diphosphates or etidronate 7.5 mg/kg/day for three days
       with steroids and IV fluids is the treatment of choice for hyper-
       calcaemia of malignancy
       Oral prednisolone (30–60 mg/day) is effective in myeloma
       and sarcoidosis   5

Chapter 4: Endocrinology Answers

Comment

Primary hyperparathyroidism may result from parathyroid adenoma (solitary adenoma accounts for over 80% of all cases), hyperplasia or carcinoma. It could occur as part of the multiple endocrine neoplasia (MEN) syndromes which are familial and inherited on a Mendelian dominant basis. Hypercalcaemic crisis is increasingly recognized as a mode of presentation of primary hyperparathyroidism in the elderly. The features are dehydration and hypotension, vomiting and fever with abdominal pains and altered level of consciousness. Emergency treatment is aimed at lowering the serum calcium. Definitive treatment is parathyroidectomy, which is performed once the patient is stable.

Answer 10   **Marks**

(a)   Phaeochromocytoma, hyperthyroidism, hypocalcaemia,
       paroxysmal atrial tachycardia, carcinoid syndrome, acute
       anxiety state   2

(b)   (i)   Phaeochromocytoma   2
       (ii)   CT scan of abdomen
       Scanning with [^{131}I] -metaiodobenzylguanidine shows
       uptake in sites of sympathetic activity. Selective venous
       sampling from renal veins for noradrenaline levels may
       be required if imaging fails to localize the lesion   3

(c)   Combined α- and β-blockade with phenoxybenzamine
       (20–40 mg/day) initially, then propranolol (120–140 mg/day)
       long term if surgical removal is not possible, or as a
       preparation for surgery, with blood transfusion to re-expand
       the contracted intra-vascular volume   3

Comment

Phaeochromocytoma is a tumour of chromaffin cells secreting catecholamines and is usually benign. It is a rare cause of hypertension and may arise from any part of the sympathetic chain but is usually found in the adrenal medulla. It should be noted that when treating with adrenergic blocking agents, beta blockade prior to alpha block may lead to hypertensive crisis, which can be fatal. In multiple endocrine neoplasia (MEN II a and b) phaeochromocytomas, usually involving both adrenal glands, are associated with medullary carcinoma of the thyroid and hyperparathyroidism, usually due to hyperplasia. In MEN type IIa, medullary carcinoma of the thyroid is associated in nearly half the patients with phaeochromocytomas, commonly bilateral, with a tendency to form phaeochromocytomas in extramedullary chromaffin tissue.

Answer 11   **Marks**

(a)   Type I diabetes mellitus   2

(b)   Raised random and fasting blood gluucose levels
       Presence of glycosuria and proteinuria
       Abnormal glucose tolerance test   4

(c)   Education about the disease – lifelong disorder
       Insulin therapy – injection method, sites, complications
       Regular blood glucose testing
       Dietary advice and review
       Stress need for compliance
       Complications viz hypo- and hyperglycaemic coma
       Wearing Medi-Alert bracelet   4

Comment

Type I diabetes mellitus is defined as a state of chronic hyperglycaemia associated with polyuria and polydypsia. In severe cases it is also associated with weight loss. The WHO criteria for diagnosing the disorder is a fasting plasma glucose of greater than 7.8 mmol/1, or a random plasma glucose of greater than 11.1 mmol/1. (In asymptomatic patients it may be necessary to obtain two such values). Patients whose plasma glucose falls between these and normal values are deemed to have impaired glucose tolerance. 2–5% of this group will become frankly diabetic and they are more prone to macrovascular complications than the normal population. Type I diabetes mellitus is now widely accepted to be an autoimmune disorder. It is thought that environmental agents trigger an immune response in genetically susceptible individuals, which leads to damage of the beta cells within the pancreas. The genetics and the mode of inheritance of the disease is extremely complex. It is thought that the racial and familial variations seen within the disease represent involvement of several different gene loci. HLA and INS (insulin) locus have both been shown to be involved. HLA DR3 and DR4 are strongly implicated in the Caucasian disease, with HLA DR2 being protective against it. Other HLA regions implicated include DQ, B8 and B15. The INS locus is on chromosome 11p. It is closely linked to a 14 base pair multiple repeat sequence which when varied in length correlates well with disease susceptiblity. Type I diabetes mellitus normally presents in young adulthood. It shows great geographical variation in incidence between 2/100,000 in Japan to 35/100,000 in areas of Scandinavia.

Answer 12   **Marks**

(a)   Hypoglycaemia
        Hyperglycaemic ketoacidosis, lactic acidosis, hyperosmolar
        non-ketotic (HONK) acidosis   2

(b)   Myocardial infarction
        Sensory neuropathy
        Nephropathy
        Recurrent infection
        Cataracts
        Peripheral vascular disease
        Diabetic retinopathy   3

(c)   Investigations –   FBC, U+Es, blood glucose
                                    Blood cultures (if indicated)
                                    CXR
                                    ECG
                                    ABGs
                                    Urinalysis – for ketones
                                    MSU
        Management –   IV access (may require central venous line)
                                    IV insulin sliding scale
                                    Treat the underlying cause, e.g. sepsis,
                                        shock, MI
                                    IV fluids – avoid dextrose until glucose is
                                        below 15 mmol/1
                                    Subcutaneous heparin (principally in
                                        HONK)   5

Comment
The recent DCCT study in the USA and the UKPDS in the United Kingdom confirmed what many doctors had believed for years: strict control of blood glucose in diabetic patients leads to fewer complications. The studies also confirmed that strict control of blood pressure [BP < 140/90] in diabetic patients was equally important. Complications may be divided into macrovascular, microvascular, neuropathic, eye and peripheral vascular disease:

- **Macrovascular** – diabetics are twice as prone to CVAs, three times more likely to have ischaemic heart disease and 50 times more likely to have a below-knee amputation compared to the normal population. Diabetic nephropathy and foot ulcers are exacerbated by macro-vascular disease.

- **Microvascular** – leads to retinopathy and nephropathy, the development of which seem to be closely linked.

- **Neuropathy** – this may be subdivided into: Peripheral sensory neuropathy – occurs in a 'glove and stocking' distribution; Autonomic neuropathy – causes postural hypotension, diarrhoea, impotence, gustatory sweating and cardiac arrhythmia; Mononeuritis multiplex – the occurrence of several individual palsies in an unrelated anatomical distribution. It may affect both the cranial and peripheral nerves; Diabetic amyotrophy – this is painful wasting and fasiculation of the quadraceps and gluteal muscles, leading to proximal lower limb weakness. The disorder is treated by placing the patient on insulin therapy which often leads to complete recovery.

- **Eye disease** – as well as retinopathy, diabetics have an increased incidence of cataracts, lipaemia retinalis, rubeosis iridis and retinal artery and venous thrombosis. It is therefore important their eyes are regularly reviewed and that worsening retinopathy or visual acuity is treated promptly by an ophthalmologist.

- **Foot disorders** – sensory neuropathy, peripheral vascular disease and microangiopathy make the feet of diabetics particularly susceptible to injury and ulceration. It is very important to emphasize good foot care, suitable footwear and supervision by a chiropodist.

CHAPTER 5: RESPIRATORY MEDICINE ANSWERS

Answer 1 Marks

(a)   To exclude a pneumothorax and consolidation/lobar collapse 2

(b)   FBC; ABGs; PEFR; blood cultures; sputum culture 3

(c) (i) Speech, pulse, respiratory rate, pulsus paradoxus,
PEFR, oxygen saturation/ABGs, cyanosis 2

   (ii) Sit the patient upright
Oxygen (60–100%) via mask; nebulized salbutamol and
ipatropium
IV access
Oral or IV steroids
Oral or IV amoxycillin +/– erythromycin 3

Comment

Asthma is defined as a reversible obstruction of the intrathoracic airways, which varies in severity either spontaneously or with treatment.

It is a common respiratory disease, affecting between 5–10% of the population. Despite the advent of several therapeutic agents including the β_2-adrenoceptor agonists, its mortality has not decreased in the last 30 years.

It is common to divide asthma into extrinsic or allergic, and intrinsic. Both groups exhibit bronchial hyperreactivity to various stimulants; these include the housedust mite, pollens, fungal spores, drugs, e.g. NSAIDs, and non-specific factors, such as emotional stress, exercise and cold air.

The severity of an acute exacerbation should be assessed by use of the following criteria.

	Mild to moderate	**Severe**
Pulse	Normal – tachycardia	Bradycardia
Blood pressure	Pulsus paradoxus	Maybe hypotensive
Respiratory rate	>25 / min	<10 / min
Speech	Normal – stilted sentences	Unable to talk
ABGs PaO$_2$	Normal to 8.0 kilopascals	<7.6–8.0 kilopascals
PaCO$_2$	Normal or low (<4.0 kilopascals)	>6.0 kilopascals
PEFR	>50% normal	<30% normal
Cyanosis	Not present	Late/sinister sign

Patients with any combination of the severe signs should be considered for elective assisted ventilation.

Answer 2   **Marks**

(a)   Atypical pneumonia   1

(b)   *Mycoplasma pneumoniae*
       Chlamydia psittaci
       Legionella pneumophila
       Coxiella burnetti   4

(c)   (i)   Haemolytic anaemia; depressed or normal WCC
              with abnormal differential count; thrombocytopaenia
       (ii)   Hyponatraemia; raised urea and creatinine
       (iii) Transient hepatitis
       (iv)   Type 1 respiratory failure
       (v)   Rising antibody titres; positive direct
              immunofluorescent stains   5

Comment

Atypical pneumonias are caused by a heterogenous group of organisms, producing atypical features compared to the pneumonias caused by Streptococcus and Haemophilus species. Some of these features are listed below:

*   **FBC** – Mycoplasma is commonly associated with a haemolytic anaemia with cold agglutinins. Legionella produces a relative lymphopaenia, whereas other organisms may depress the white cell count to subnormal levels. Many of the atypical organisms may also produce a thrombocytopenia.
*   **U+Es** – SIADH producing a hyponatraemia is a feature of several atypicals, particularly Legionella infection. Dehydration, secondary to nausea and vomiting or diarrhoea, may cause mild pre-renal impairment.
*   **LFTs** – A transient hepatitis is another common feature which may, in turn, be exacerbated by erythromycin.
*   **Skin** – Generalized rashes are common but Mycoplasma may cause erythema multiforme and the Stevens–Johnson syndrome. *Chlamydia psittaci* may cause rose spots on the abdomen.
*   **CNS** – Drowsiness and confusion may be features, as may depression. They may also present with a meningitic picture, as well as causing a meningo-encephalitis.

Other features include diarrhoea and vomiting, pharyngitis and more unusually pericarditis, myocarditis and rarely Coxiella-associated endocarditis. The organisms are generally difficult to culture in the laboratory but are now more readily identifiable by use of direct immunofluorescent stains and specific antibodies. Treatment may include the use of erythromycin, tetracycline, and rifampicin, but should always include anti-streptococcal agents, as it is far more common, and can be fatal if untreated.

Answer 3   **Marks**

(a)   A full respiratory and cardiovascular history
       Previous medical history – particularly previous whooping
       cough, measles, asthma, tuberculosis
       Treatment history to exclude exacerbating drugs, e.g. NSAIDs
       and beta-blockers
       Smoking history – duration, type, number/day
       Occupational history – e.g. exposure to industrial dusts
       Exposure to domestic animals and birds   5

(b)   Chest X-ray, PEFR, spirometery – pre and post nebulizer,
       ECG, ABGs   3

(c) β_2-agonists – salbutamol, terbutaline
       Anticholinergics – ipatropium bromide
       Theophylline – aminophylline
       Steroids – inhaled, oral or intravenous   2

Comment
By definition chronic bronchitis is a clinical diagnosis, based on a productive cough for three or more months in two or more consecutive years. Emphysema is a pathological diagnosis, and is defined as dilatation and destruction of the airways distal to the terminal bronchioles. Both may produce a similar clinical picture, which is classically divided into the 'pink puffer' and the 'blue bloater', suffering type 1 and type 2 failure, respectively. Type I respiratory failure is defined as hypoxia (PaO_2<10.6 kilopascals) associated with a normal or low arterial carbon dioxide, ($PaCO_2$ = 4.6 kilopascals), whereas type II failure is hypoxia associated with a raised arterial carbon dioxide ($PaCO_2$>6.4 kilopascals). Therapeutic agents such as β_2-agonists, anticholinergics, theophylline and steroids are often given with subjective improvement, but no interventions other than cessation of smoking and long term oxygen therapy have any bearing on prognosis. Patients qualify for long term home oxygen by fulfilling the following criteria, based on two sets of arterial blood gases and spirometry, with the patient stable: PaO_2 <7.3 kilopascals; $PaCO_2$ >6.0 kilopascals; FEV <1.5 litres; FVC <2.0 litres.

Morbidity is reduced if patients wear their oxygen appliance for 15–19 hours per day; mortality being reduced when worn for >19 hours per day.

Answer 4   **Marks**

(a)   Bronchogenic carcinoma   1

(b)   CXR; sputum for cytology; bronchoscopy with brushings
        and biopsy
        CT scan of the thorax   3

(c)   Chemotherapy is used alone or as an adjuvant to surgery
        and/or radiotherapy
        Surgery – may be curative; may be combined with chemo-
        therapy and radiotherapy
        Radiotherapy – may be used as a monotherapy or in
        combination. It is also used to palliate bony pain of
        metastases and for recurrent haemoptysis
        Palliative care involving specialist medical and nursing
        staff should be considered in cases presenting with
        advanced disease   6

Comment
Bronchial carcinoma is the commonest malignancy in the Western world, with an annual mortality of 35,000 people in the UK alone. It affects 3–4 times as many men as women, but the female incidence continues to increase. In this case the diagnosis of carcinoma is the most likely, although pulmonary tuberculosis, bronchiectasis, lung abscess and the systemic vasculitides may all present in this way. The diagnosis may be inferred from a chest X-ray and confirmed by sputum cytology and bronchoscopy with bronchial washings and biopsy. CT scan of the thorax may be required to localize and stage the tumour. The therapeutic options include surgery, chemotherapy, radiotherapy, and palliative care. Operative intervention is limited by the patient's respiratory reserve, the anatomical site and staging of the tumour. However, in non-small cell disease, it is potentiallly curative. In general, elderly patients do badly with surgery. Chemotherapy is principally used in small cell disease, where it is proven to improve prognosis. Combination therapy is now also used in advanced, inoperable non-small cell disease, but with little effect on long term prognosis. Various combinations of chemotherapeutic agents are used, including adriamycin, methotrexate, cyclophosphamide and newer agents, including ifosfamide.

Answer 5   **Marks**

(a)   Pulmonary embolism   1

(b)   Recent long distance journey or prolonged period of
       immobility
       Recent major surgery
       Recent fracture – particularly pelvic and lower limb
       Family history of coagulopathy or thromboembolic disease
       Oral contraceptive pill and pregnancy
       Coagulopathy – Protein C and S, anti-thrombin III
       deficiency; anticardiolipin antibody; Factor V Leiden
       Malignancy   3

(c)   (i)   Investigations –
                     FBC, clotting screen
                     ABGs
                     CXR
                     ECG
                     V/Q scan or pulmonary angiography   3
       (ii)   Therapeutic management
              Sit the patient upright; oxygen via a mask
              IV access
              Analgesia
              Intravenous or subcutaneous heparin (20–40,000
              units/24hours, depending on the weight of the patient)
              On confirmation of the diagnosis, 6 months' therapy
              with warfarin, maintaining the INR between 2–3
              Address and treat underlying risk factors   3

Comment
One should always have a low threshold for treating a patient for pulmonary
embolism, particularly in the presence of any combination of risk factors. (A
second embolism could be fatal!) Initial investigations may often produce
non-specific results but add to clinical suspicions:
*   **FBC** – this may show polycythaemia, thrombocytosis or an abnormal
    white cell count suggestive of a haematological malignancy.
*   **Clotting screen** – in cases where there is no identifiable risk factors
    this should include protein C and S, and anti-thrombin III levels, and
    anticardiolipin antibody. Recently, Factor V Leiden deficiency has
    been identified as an important cause in this subgroup.

- **ABGs** – show type I respiratory failure, often with hypocapnia.
- **ECG** – the principal abnormality is a sinus tachycardia, but in larger PEs a right ventricular strain pattern may occur, with a dominant R wave in V1 and V2. The classical pattern of S1Q3T3 is rarely seen, but should always be sought.
- **CXR** – may be normal, however, it may produce a wedge shadow or oligaemic areas. It is also necessary to exclude pneumonias and pneumothoraces, which may present in a similar manner.

Definitive investigations include a V/Q (ventilation/perfusion) scan, but this may be limited, particularly when there is underlying pulmonary disease. Pulmonary angiography remains the 'gold standard', but is rarely used in general hospital practice.

Answer 6   **Marks**

(a)   Erythema nodosum
         Keratoconjunctivitis sicca   2

(b)   Skin involvement – lupus pernio, sarcoid infiltration of the skin
         Neurological – peripheral neuropathy, cranial nerve palsies,
                   aseptic meningitis, hypopituitarism
         Eyes – anterior uveitis, choroidoretinitis
         'Sicca syndrome' – infiltration of the salivary and lacrimal
                   glands
         Joints – arthralgia
         Hepatosplenomegaly
         Renal – renal stones, hypercalciuria and associated
                   nephrocalcinosis
         Lymphadenopathy
         Cardiomyopathy, cor pulmonale and conduction system
                   disease   3

(c)   CXR
         Transbronchial biopsy and broncho-alveolar lavage
         Liver biopsy
         Formal respiratory function tests
         Serum angiotensin converting enzyme (ACE)
         Kveim test
         Tuberculin test   5

Comment

Sarcoidosis is a common, multisystem granulomatous disorder, which presents usually between 25–35 years of age. It is more common in women and in certain racial groups. It has a more severe presentation and malignant progression in Black compared to Caucasian races. Clinically it is characterized by pulmonary infiltration, skin and eye involvement, and on chest X-ray by bilateral hilar lymphadenopathy. The pathogenesis and aetiology remain unclear. It is thought that environmental agents trigger an abnormal immune response, with helper T-cells at its centre. These cause the formation of non-caseating granulomata, which in turn leads to a fibrotic response in the affected tissues. The course and prognosis of the disease can be inferred by the mode of presentation. Acute onset in young adults, with associated erythema nodosum, usually signifies a self-limiting disorder. Later, more insidious onset in middle age leads to a progressive disorder, with multisystem fibrosis.

Pulmonary sarcoid is classified by the radiological changes seen on chest X-ray, into four stages:

- Stage 0 (clear CXR)
- Stage 1 (bilateral hilar and mediastinal lymphadenopathy)
- Stage 2 (stage 1 + associated pulmonary infiltration)
- Stage 3 (pulmonary infiltration without hilar lymphadenopathy)

No therapy has as yet been shown to influence the progression of the disease. Steroids are recomended in stages 2 and 3 of the pulmonary disease, and for eye and cardiac involvement. Chloroquine is also used in therapy, as are NSAIDs.

Answer 7   **Marks**

(a)   Cystic fibrosis   1

(b)   Pancreatic endocrine involvement leading to diabetes mellitus
       Pancreatic exocrine involvement leading to steatorrhoea and
       malabsorption
       Bronchiectasis   3

(c)   Nutritional support with pancreatic enzyme supplements and
       regular dietetic review
       Diabetic education and insulin therapy
       Daily chest physiotherapy, which may be performed by
       relatives

    Rapid and appropiate treatment of infective exacerbations
    Sputum viscosity reduction
    Genetic counselling of parents and patient
    Consider for heart lung transplant   6

Comment

Cystic fibrosis is an autosomal recessive disorder, whose gene mutation has now been localized to the long arm of chromosome 7. The protein encoded in this region is called the cystic fibrosis transmembrane regulator. With improvements in physiotherapy, antimicrobials and nutritional support, life expectancy in this group has now improved to 30–40 years. Patients usually present in childhood with recurrent pulmonary symptoms, cystic fibrosis being the principal cause of chronic suppurative lung disease in this age group. They may also present with constipation or even acute obstruction due to meconium ileus equivalent (MIE), meconium ileus being a presenting feature in the neonate.

Males are invariably infertile due to the absence of development of the vas deferens and the epididymus, but females are able to conceive providing the secondary effects of the illness, such as malnutrition, can be prevented or minimized.

The diagnosis is confirmed from the family history, a sodium sweat test and chromosomal analysis. Treatment should be instituted and followed up in a regional or area centre of excellence, so that complications of the disease are rapidly identified and minimised. Pseudomonal chest infection is the main cause of exacerbation of the chest symptoms and is often the cause of death. Newer anti-pseudomonal agents have recently been developed, including ticarcillin, azlocillin, imipenim, tobramycin and ciprofloxacin. Providing the patient's health can be stabilized, there is 65% survival at three years and 50% survival at five years. In severe cases a heart–lung transplant remains the only viable option at the present time. Gene manipulation may offer a future cure.

Answer 8   **Marks**

(a)   Cryptogenic fibrosing alveolitis   1

(b)   Rheumatoid arthritis, systemic lupus erythrematosus
        Progressive systemic sclerosis
        Inflammatory bowel disease
        Primary biliary cirrhosis   3

(c)   CXR – lower zone fibrosis

ABGs – type I respiratory failure
Lung function tests – restrictive lung defect, with a reduced
    transfer coefficient
High resolution CT scan of the thorax – confirms the
    distribution of the fibrosis   6

Comment

Cryptogenic fibrosing alveolitis is defined as fibrosis of the distal airways, in
the absence of any identifiable cause. It may present at any age but is most
commonly seen in the sixth and seventh decades. It has an equal sex
distribution but its prevalence is increased amongst smokers. It is associated
with several immune mediated disorders, but its own aetiology remains
unclear. Patients present with progressive exertional dyspnoea, associated
with a non-productive cough. Haemoptysis is a sinister sign and should alert
the physician to the possibility of an underlying malignancy, which is 10–15
times more common than in the general population. Clubbing occurs in
70–80% of cases and many also have fine inspiratory crepitations, principally
heard at the lung bases. In the more severe cases, there may also be cyanosis
and signs of cor pulmonale. The diagnosis is confirmed by lung function tests,
high resolution CT scan of the thorax, and bronchoscopy and broncho-
alveolar lavage. Arterial blood gases show type I respiratory failure, the
hypoxia classically worsening on exertion. Since the disease is idiopathic,
there is no specific treatment. Various new regimes are under investigation,
including high dose steroids, and immunosuppressents, such as azothioprine,
cyclophosphamide and cyclosporin, but the prognosis remains poor with a
50% mortality at five years.

Answer 9   **Marks**

(a)   The pneumoconioses
       Silicosis
       Berylliosis   3

(b)   His shortness of breath is caused by pulmonary fibrosis
       secondary to asbestosis. The haemoptysis is secondary to a
       bronchogenic carcinoma   2

(c)   Pleural thickening
       Calcified pleural and diaphragmatic plaques
       Lower zone fibrosis initially, which may become more widespread
       Advanced cases may show signs of 'honeycombing', with a

hazy irregular cardiac silhouette
Bronchial carcinoma and associated signs, e.g. hilar
lymphadenopathy   5

Comment
Chronic exposure to asbestos, in particular, crocidolite (blue asbestos) causes
a chronic pulmonary fibrotic disorder, asbestosis. This classically affects the
lower zones of the lungs, unlike the other pneumoconioses, which affect the
apices. (The radiological findings of pleural and diaphragmatic plaques only
imply previous asbestos exposure and the patient should not be labelled as
having asbestosis.)
Asbestos exposure is the principal risk factor in the development of
mesothelioma, which may be pleural, peritoneal and more rarely pericardial.
Both the duration and the concentration of fibre exposure are important in the
development of the tumour. Classically the tumour manifests itself 30–40
years after the initial exposure. There is currently no effective treatment and
the prognosis remains poor, with a median survival of 18 months. Smoking
has a synergistic effect with asbestos fibres and increases the risk of developing a bronchogenic carcinoma almost 100 times that of a non-smoker never
exposed to asbestos.
Asbestosis and the other pneumoconioses are industrial notifiable diseases in
the UK, for which the patient and their families are eligible for compensation.

Answer 10   **Marks**

(a)   Farmer's lung; this is an example of extrinsic allergic alveolitis 2
(c)   He should be advised:

(b)
Agents	Sources	
Aspergillus Spp	whisky maltings, vegetable compost	
Penicillium Spp	cheese, wood, cork	
Birds	feathers and excreta	4

Chronic exposure may cause a progressive lung condition with
fibrosis, causing increasing shortness of breath and disability;
minimize exposure to precipitating agents by changing his
work duties, using an industrial respirator to filter out dusts,
and improve the ventilation in the working environment;
the use of oral and inhaled steroids is beneficial in an acute
attack   4

Comment
Extrinsic allergic alveolitis is the term given to the group of pulmonary disorders caused by hypersensitivity to inhaled dusts. They are alternatively termed hypersensitivity pneumonitis, as the resulting inflammatory process occurs in all of the distal airways involved in gaseous exchange, and not just the alveoli.

Clinically the disease is divided into acute and chronic forms. In the **acute form** the sensitized patient, i.e. someone previously exposed to the causative dust, presents several hours after a further exposure, with acute dyspnoea and a non-productive cough. They often complain of an associated flu-like illness. Occasionally, the patient may present with a wheeze and a productive cough predominating. In the **chronic form** there is progressive pulmonary fibrosis, principally in the apices of the lungs. As the diseases progresses the fibrosis becomes more widespread and this leads to secondary pulmonary hypertension and cor pulmonale.

Management is based on excluding or reducing exposure to the causative agent. However, patients often chose to continue exposure, e.g. pigeon fanciers. In industrial cases the patient is eligible for compensation if the chronic form of the disease develops, but many patients with the acute form choose to continue working, with few progressing to the chronic, symptomatic disease. In these cases inhaled or oral steroids are used in acute on chronic episodes, however, the use of long term steroids in the chronic disease has not been shown to influence the prognosis.

Answer 11   **Marks**

(a)   Adult respiratory distress syndrome (ARDS)   1

(b)   CXR appearances of pulmonary oedema
          Hypoxaemia (PaO_2 < 6.7 kilopascals), on 60–100%
          inspired oxygen   2

(c)   (i)   FBC, U+Es, glucose, clotting screen including
                  FDPs and D-dimer, group and save
              Blood cultures
              ABGs
              CXR
              ECG
              MSU or CSU   3

    (ii)   Management is based on the haemodynamic
               status of the patient:

With adequate blood pressure – sit the patient upright
If the patient is shocked – start colloid infusion
Patient will require central venous access and inotrope
support, therefore more senior help should be
sought immediately
In either case –

Intravenous access
60–100% oxygen via a mask
IV broad spectrum antibiotics and diuretics   4

Comment

ARDS should always be suspected in any patient with acute respiratory failure and any predisposing factors, such as:

Hypovolaemia/haemorrhage
Sepsis – this is implicated in 80% of cases
Trauma – this includes burns
Thrombotic, fat and amniotic emboli
Aspiration pneumonia and drowning
Inhalation of smoke and noxious gases
Drug overdose – barbiturates, NSAIDs, heroin
Metabolic disturbances – uraemia, ketoacidosis

ARDS has several diagnostic criteria:

CXR – the radiographic changes vary from isolated areas to diffuse alveolar infiltration, consistent with pulmonary oedema; they often correlate poorly with the clinical condition of the patient
Hypoxaemia – the PaO_2 must be <6.7 kilopascals on 60–100% inspired oxygen
Reduced lung compliance – this is confirmed on ventilating the patient
Exudative pulmonary oedema
PCWP<18 mm Hg – this excludes cardiogenic oedema, where the PCWP is >18 mm Hg
Pulmonary hypertension > 30/15 mm Hg

Treatment should include appropiate management of the underlying cause, correction of any specific metabolic disturbances and assisted ventilation in an intensive care unit. No specific treatment has been shown to influence the prognosis. Failure to recognise and treat the condition leads to rapid deposition of proteinaceous and hyaline material leading to alveolar collapse and, within 48 hours, irreversible interstitial fibrosis.

CHAPTER 6: CARDIOLOGY ANSWERS

Answer 1   **Marks**

(a) (i) Acute myocardial infarction   1

    (ii) Risk factors – smoking
        Previous history of IHD or CVA
        Known diabetes mellitus, hypertension, PVD
        Family history of IHD or CVA   2

(b)   Aspirin
        Beta-blockers, e.g. atenolol, metoprolol
        ACEIs, e.g. captopril, enalapril, ramipril, lisinopril, perindopril
        Thrombolytic agents, e.g. streptokinase, tPA
        Lipid lowering agents, e.g. privastatin, simvastatin
        Insulin   3

(c)   History – need to clarify site, character, time of onset,
                duration, intensity/severity, radiation of the pain
                exacerbating/relieving factors, risk factors, present
                medications, contraindications to thrombolysis
    Examination – assess haemodynamic status, signs of
                cardiac failure, presence of murmurs, signs of
                hyperlipidaemia, PVD, hypertension, diabetes mellitus
    Investigations –   FBC, U+Es, glucose, lipids, cardiac
                            enzymes
                            CXR
                            ECG
    Treatment –   Sit the patient upright, IV access
                  Oxygen via a mask, analgesia
                  Aspirin 300 mg (stat)
                  Confirm diagnosis based on history,
                  examination, ECG, and cardiac enzymes
                  If no contraindications give thrombolysis
    In next 24–48 hours consider secondary prophylaxis, i.e.
    ACEIs and/or beta-blockers; address all risk factors;
    education re: lifestyle by specialist nurse practitioners   4

Comment

Within the last 15 years, several worldwide mega trials, in particular the ISIS series and GUSTO, have dramatically changed the treatment and prognosis of acute myocardial infarction. Aspirin, thrombolysis, and insulin have all been shown to improve prognosis in the first 24 hours, and secondary prophylaxis with ACEIs, beta-blockers and simvastatin have improved post-infarction morbidity and survival.

Admission of a patient with a confirmed infarct can be divided into two phases: the acute phase or first 24 hours and the secondary phase, which incorporates the rest of the admission and beyond.

Acute phase:

* Diagnosis is confirmed by history, examination, and investigations
* Sit the patient upright, oxygen via mask
* IV access
* Analgesia – initially sublingual or buccal nitrates
  If this has poor effect, IV diamorphine with IV anti-emetic is given (drugs should not be administered IM as this will affect the enzyme results)
* Stat dose of aspirin 300 mg

If no contraindications the patient should receive thrombolysis. tPA should be given in patients presenting early (less than four hours after onset of symptoms), with an anterior MI. In all other cases, streptokinase remains the first line choice in the UK. The patient should be admitted to CCU, and should have serial enzymes and ECGs.

(Secondary phase treatment and prophylaxis is dealt with in the next question.)

Patients with Non Q wave infarcts (previously known as subendocardial infarcts) or unstable angina should receive aspirin, low molecular weight subcutaneous heparin, and nitrates to control pain. GII_B/III_a receptor antagonists are also approved for use in such patients.

Answer 2   **Marks**

(a)   Aspirin
       ACE inhibitor
       Lipid lowering agent, e.g. simvastatin
       Oral hypoglycaemic, e.g. gliclazide   4

(b)   Dietitian – needs advice on low cholesterol, diabetic diet   1

(c)   Address all risk factors – hyperlipidaemia, diabetes, smoking,
       alcohol excess, obesity, lack of exercise
       Patient education about prognosis and lifestyle
       Education about further angina, the possible need for anti-
       anginal therapy and the use of GTN tablets or spray; if regular
       chest pain, he will require further investigation, which includes
       exercise stress testing and possible coronary angiography   5

Comment

All patients suffering from ischaemic heart disease should be on some form of secondary prophylaxis. Patients with no contraindications should be on low dose aspirin, 75 mg per day, and depending on their left ventricular function, a beta-blocker or an ACE inhibitor, and in some cases both. Left ventricular function is assessed clinically, by the presence or absence of basal crepitations, radiographically, by the CXR signs of pulmonary oedema and cardiomegaly, and objectively by echocardiography. ACE inhibitors stop 'ventricular remodelling' which occurs after an ischaemic insult, thus reducing 'dysfunctional contractility' of the affected myocardium. Beta-blockers reduce the myocardial contractility and therefore reduce the demand for increased blood supply. Recent work has shown that ACE inhibitors improve the prognosis in all patients, irrespective of their left ventricular function, and that in patients with mild to moderate left ventricular impairment, beta-blockers should now be given with or without an ACE inhibitor. In practice, however, most patients are placed on only one of these agents. On-going anginal symptoms require medical intervention with antianginal therapy. Beta-blockers are the first line choice, if not contra-indicated, then depending on symptoms, oral nitrates, calcium channel blockers and potassium channel activators, can be added. If medical therapy fails to control anginal symptoms further investigations should be initiated, starting with an exercise stress test. The patient must be made aware that depending on the results of this test, they may require coronary angiography, angioplasty or possible bypass surgery.

Answer 3   **Marks**

(a)   Beta-blockers and calcium channel blockers   2

(b)   The radiological features include:
        Cardiomegaly, upper lobe blood diversion, Kerley B lines,
        pleural effusions, fluid in the horizontal fissure, and interstitial
        shadowing consistent with pulmonary oedema
        Other findings may include –
            calcification of the heart valves
            left ventricular aneurysm   4

(c)   Management should include:
        Full history and examination to identify underlying risk
        factors and their associated signs

Investigations –	FBC, U+Es, glucose, lipids, TFTs
	CXR
	ECG
	echocardiogram

Address any underlying risk factors: stop smoking, decrease
alcohol excess, improve diet, weight loss if appropriate – review
by dietitian, hypertension, hyperlipidaemia, unstable angina
Increase exercise participation
Specific therapeutic agents – diuretics, ACE inhibitors,
digoxin, nitrates, others, e.g. hydralazine   4

Comment

The prognosis in biventricular cardiac failure remains poor, despite the introduction of new therapeutic agents such as ACE inhibitors. The one-year
mortality is approximately 50%. Ischaemic heart disease, hypertension and
idiopathic dilated cardiomyopathy remain by far the commonest causes in the
Western world. Others include:

- Cardiomyopathy (toxic, e.g. alcohol)
- Restrictive
- Hypertrophic
- Myocardial infiltration (fibrosis, sarcoidosis, amyloidosis,
  haemochromatosis)
- Valvular dysfunction (endocarditis, rheumatic valvular disease,
  congenital valvular disease)
- Chronic arrhythmia (brady and tachyarrhythmia)
- Drugs (beta-blockers, NSAIDs, calcium channel blockers)
- Systemic disease (acromegaly, thyroid disease, anaemia)

The management of heart failure must initially address any underlying risk
factors, associated disease, and improve the patients understanding of their
condition.

First line medications should include loop diuretics and ACE inhibitors, and then
with symptom progression, nitrates, digoxin and vasodilators, such as prazosin,
should be introduced. Formal anticoagulation should also be considered, as this
group are particularly at risk from DVT and left ventricular thrombus formation.
Cardiac transplant although offering a 'cure', remains limited due to lack of
donor hearts and financial constraint. Transplant survival is estimated at 50%
at five years. Trials with implantable mechanical pumps are underway.

Answer 4   Marks

(a) (i) Atrial fibrillation   1

    (ii) Ischaemic heart disease – due to smoking and alcohol excess

Cardiomyopathy – due to alcohol excess or ischaemic
heart disease   2

(b)   Transient ischaemic attack   2

(c)   History and examination – to assess risk factors and their
       associated signs in particular hypertension, cardiac murmurs,
       and cardiac failure
       Investigations –   FBC, U+Es, glucose, lipids, TFTs
                                 CXR
                                 ECG
                                 24-hour tape
                                 Echocardiogram
       Therapeutic management:
               Address underlying risk factors and associated disease
               Drugs – digoxin, amiodarone, sotalol
               Add aspirin 300 mg o.d. in this case (alcohol excess
               precludes formal anticoagulation with warfarin)
               Consider synchronized DC cardioversion   5

Comment
Atrial fibrillation, particularly in its paroxysmal form, is associated with
increased morbidity and mortality. Systemic emboli lead to TIAs, CVAs,
limb and mesenteric embolization, all of which may be fatal. Once the
diagnosis is confirmed, the aim of therapy is to cardiovert the patient back
into sinus rhythm, which maybe achieved either chemically with drugs or by
synchronized DC cardioversion. If this is unachievable then control of the
ventricular rate must be achieved by drug therapy. The patient should be
anticoagulated with warfarin, with the INR kept between 2–3. If warfarin is
contraindicated then aspirin should be considered. Once the patient has been
anticoagulated for at least three weeks, synchronized DC cardioversion
maybe attempted. However, it is rarely used in patients with chronic organic
heart disease or longstanding arrhythmia, as the success rate is poor. Medical
therapy should be instituted in all patients with confirmed arrhythmia.
Digoxin or amiodarone form the basis of most patients' therapy, although
sotalol is now recommended in patients with good residual left ventricular
function. Amiodarone is an extremely useful antidysrrhythmic but it has
numerous side effects of which the patient must be made aware. These
include:
•   Skin (slate grey pigmentation and photosensitivity)
•   Pulmonary fibrosis (this is rare in doses below 400 mg per day)

- Thyroid dysfunction (it may cause both hyper- and hypothyroidism)
- Hepatitis

It is important therefore to have baseline LFTs, TFTs, and pulmonary function tests, and to record that the patient has been made aware of the possible side effects.

Answer 5   **Marks**

(a) (i) Infective endocarditis   1
   (ii) Osler's nodes – painful, red indurating lesions in the finger
      pulps
      Janeway lesions – macular, non-tender lesions on the palm
      and soles
      Roth spots – retinal haemorrhages with pale, exudative
      centres   3

(b) Two to three sets of blood cultures before starting antibiotics
    Echocardiogram   2

(c) Cardiovascular –   cardiac failure, pericarditis
                aortic root abscess
                haemolytic anaemia
    Systemic –   meningitis, meningo-encephalitis
                mycotic aneurysms
                left-sided valves – systemic emboli
                right-sided valves – pulmonary emboli
                renal failure   4

Comment

Infective endocarditis may present in an acute or chronic manner, the acute form often running a malignant course. Although there are many people potentially at risk in the general population, the advent of antibiotics and the reduction in incidence of rheumatic valvular disease has meant the pattern and outcome of the disease has changed for the better over the century. The disease is now more prevalent in men and is becoming increasingly prevalent in the elderly population. However, despite the improvements in prognosis, the acute form, particularly when caused by *Staphylococcus aureus* and *Streptococcus pneumoniae* infections, still carries a 30% mortality.

Common causative organisms include:

- Streptococci (viridans, milleri, bovis, sanguis and mutans)
- Staphylococci (aureus, epidermidis, hominis)

- Gram-negative organisms
- Pseudomonas
- HACEK group (Haemophilus Spp, Actinobacillus, *Actinomyces comitans*, *Cardiobacterium hominis*, *Eikenella corrodens*, *Kingella kingae*)

Rarer organisms include *Coxiella burnetti*, Brucella, Klebsiella, *E. coli*. Any patient presenting with signs of sepsis and a cardiac murmur should alert the clinician to possible endocarditis. In the elderly it is always a diagnosis to exclude, as it often presents in a non-specific manner. Blood cultures are positive in 90–95% of cases, and attempts should be made to obtain two to three sets in the hour before commencing antibiotic therapy. Echocardiography is the only other specific investigation, and is also quite sensitive. In patients where aortic root disease is suspected transoesophageal echo should be considered. Empirical treatment is often used in the severely sick or acute presentation, and consists of intravenous penicillin and gentamicin. If Staphylococcus is suspected then flucloxacillin may be added.

Answer 6   **Marks**

(a)   Hypertrophic obstructive cardiomyopathy (HOCM)
       Autosomal dominant   2

(b)   Ischaemic heart disease, hypertension, alcohol, sarcoidosis   3

(c)   Investigations –   resting ECG; 48-hour tape
                              CXR
                              Echocardiogram with Doppler
                              Exercise testing with continuous BP
                              monitoring
       Medical therapy – amiodarone, beta-blockers, calcium
       channel blockers
       Surgical intervention – resection of outflow tract
       In familial cases such as this, sibling and children screening   5

Comment

HOCM is an idiopathic disorder, which is usually familial, and is inherited in an autosomal dominant manner. Recent work using chromosomal analysis of families with the disease have identified abnormalities in the genes for troponin, myosin and tropomyosin. Clinically, patients present with symptoms of ventricular outflow tract obstruction, or tachyarrhythmia. Chest pain, dyspnoea, palpitations and syncope are common, but there may be few symptoms prior to sudden death. Examination is often unremarkable, but may reveal signs of left or right ventricular outflow tract obstruction and associated dysfunction, which is commoner in younger patients. The classical murmur associated with HOCM is mid-systolic, and is accompanied by a forceful apex beat and a fourth heart sound. The intensity of the murmur is increased with exercise. Investigation is aimed at identifying the subgroup of patients with non-sustained ventricular tachycardia (VT), which has the greatest bearing on prognosis and, in particular, the likelihood of sudden death. Therefore essential investigations must include a 48-hour tape. Echocardiography with colour Doppler flow has recently superseded angiography in the younger patient. It can be used to assess not only the left ventricular dimensions and function but also the outflow tract. Cardiac catheter studies are now principally reserved for patients over the age of 40 to assess the coronary circulation. Specific therapy in those with non-sustained VT should include amiodarone. Propranolol and verapamil are also used. Patients with outflow tract gradients greater than 50 mm Hg, should be considered for surgical resection. The role of permanent pacemakers is still being evaluated.

Answer 7   **Marks**

(a) Fallot's tetralogy
     Eisenmenger's syndrome (right to left shunt across a
     ventricular septal defect)
     Transposition of the great vessels   3

(b) Right ventricular outflow tract obstruction – usually
     pulmonary valvular stenosis
     Ventricular septal defect, with an overriding aorta
     Right ventricular hypertrophy   4

(c) Surgical repair is the only curative treatment. It is usually
     divided into two procedures
     (i)   palliative shunt formation, followed 6 months to 1 year
           later by
     (ii) complete repair
     In patients presenting with advanced disease – palliation with
     diuretics and oxygen   3

Comment
Patients who undergo surgical correction for Fallot's tetralogy generally do very well, and go on to live normal lives. With advances in obstetric antenatal

imaging and paediatric screening, most cases are picked up early and few now present with advanced disease. Initial surgical correction involves the formation of a palliative shunt between the pulmonary and systemic vasculature. This is particularly important when pulmonary atresia or severe polycythaemia is present. The aim of the shunt is to increase blood flow through the pulmonary vasculature and the left side of the heart. The shunts used are:

- Blalock (subclavian artery to either pulmonary artery)
- Waterston (ascending thoracic aorta to the right pulmonary artery)
- Potts (descending thoracic aorta to the left pulmonary artery)

Women who have had any congenital heart defect are at greater risk of having children with heart defects and therefore must be carefully monitored with foetal echocardiography throughout their pregnancy.

Answer 8   **Marks**

(a)   Acute left ventricular failure – this is the most likely diagnosis
        Tachyarrhythmia – atrial fibrillation, ventricular tachycardia
        or fibrillation
        Reinfarction
        Asthma
        Bronchospasm secondary to beta-blockade
        Pulmonary embolism   3

(b)   FBC, U+Es, glucose, cardiac enzymes (CK and AST)
        CXR
        ECG
        ABGs   3

(c)   Sit the patient upright
        Oxygen via face mask
        IV access
        IV frusemide 40–80 mg + / – IV diamorphine and antiemetic
        If severe consider – IV nitrate infusion and urinary catheter
        Monitor BP, pulse, oxygen saturation, cardiac monitor
        If haemodynamically compromised – will need central venous
        line and inotrope support   4

Comment

Left ventricular failure is a common complication of acute myocardial infarction. It may be precipitated by:

- Reinfarction or ongoing unstable angina

- Acute mitral regurgitation ⎱ Both may be inferred by a new
- Acute ventricular septal defect ⎰ pansystolic murmur
- Haemopericardium or acute ventricular rupture
- Arrhythmia (AF, SVT, VF or VT, complete heart block and bradyarrhythmia)
- Beta-blockade with existing impaired left ventricular function

Acute therapy is largely dependent on the haemodynamic status of the patient. If the patient is maintaining a reasonable blood pressure (>100 mm Hg systolic) then IV loop diuretics and then IV nitrates should be employed which 'off-load' the heart. Intravenous diamorphine may also be used. This acts as an anxiolytic, but also has local pulmonary effects. All of these treatments cause hypotension, and it is therefore important to monitor the patient at all times. Patients who are haemodynamically compromised should have a central venous line and urinary catheter inserted, to monitor fluid balance. They will also require inotrope support with dobutamine and in severe cases adrenaline and noradrenaline. Underlying factors, such as arrhythmia, need to be treated and mechanical problems, such as acute ventricular septal defect or mitral regurgitation, require surgical intervention.

Answer 9   **Marks**

(a) (i) Aortic stenosis   1
   (ii) Congenital bicuspid valve
     Rheumatic valvular disease   2

(b)   Slow rising pulse
     Narrow pulse pressure
     Non-displaced heaving apex beat
     Ejection systolic murmur, radiating to the carotids   3

(c)   Investigations – CXR, ECG, echocardiogram, cardiac
     catheter studies
     Management – aortic valve replacement (unless medically unfit) 4

Comment

Aortic stenosis is a common valvular disorder, primarily caused by degenerative change in a congenitally bicuspid valve. The commonest acquired cause remains rheumatic valvular disease. Clinically the patient presents with symptoms of left ventricular dysfunction and outflow tract obstruction. In significant disease this usually manifests itself as exertional angina, pulmonary oedema, and exertional syncope. It may also cause sudden death.

Examination of the patient will reveal a slow rising pulse with a low volume. The pulse pressure is narrow. The apex beat is non-displaced and is hyper-dynamic or 'heaving' in nature. On auscultation there is an ejection systolic murmur which radiates to the carotids. The aortic component of the second heart sound maybe soft or absent with reverse splitting of this sound. There may also be a fourth heart sound, and an ejection click. All patients require both echocardiography and cardiac catheter studies, the latter to assess both the gradient across the valve, and the coronary circulation. Surgical replacement of the valve is the only curative treatment. Diuretic therapy maybe instituted in the inoperable or acute presentation, but should not be prolonged if surgery is being contemplated as it may exacerbate the condition.

Answer 10   **Marks**

(a)   FBC, U+Es, glucose, lipids
        Urinalysis – protein, blood, glucose
        CXR
        ECG   2

(b)   Diuretics – bendrofluazide
        Beta-blockers – atenolol, oxprenolol
        Calcium channel blockers – diltiazem, verapamil, nifedipine,
        amlodipine, lacidipine
        ACEI – lisinopril, perindopril
        Alpha blockers – doxazosin
        Angiotensin II Antagonists – volsartan, candesartan,
        irbesartan   4

(c)   Address all risk factors –
                smoking, alcohol excess, obesity, lack of exercise,
                diabetes mellitus, hyperlipidaemia (these will need to
                reviewed by a dietitian and specialist diabetic liaison
                nurse)
        Institute medical therapy – tailored to the individual patient   4

Comment
Essential or primary hypertension is responsible for 90–95% of all cases of hypertensive disease. It is a complex multifactorial disorder, which arises due to interactions of genetic and environmental factors. Several genes in combination predispose an individual to develop hypertension, but it is exposure to various environmental factors which determines expression and

progression of the disease. These factors include:

- **Diet** – various components of our diet have been related to the development of hypertension. Excess sodium and low potassium intake have both been postulated, but there remains limited evidence to support this. Vegetarians have lower blood pressure than their age-matched omnivorous counterparts, but this may also be multifactorial
- **Obesity** – this involves neuroendocrine dysfunction and environ-mental factors such as lack of exercise
- **Alcohol excess** – greater than six units of alcohol per day is known to cause hypertension. Conversely, reduction in alcohol intake will lower the blood pressure
- **Environmental stress** – although this is known to cause acute rises in blood pressure, its long term effects remain unknown
- **Lack of exercise** – improving exercise participation not only lowers blood pressure, it also improves prognosis in other related cardiovascular disease, e.g. biventricular cardiac failure. All of these risk factors, as well as diabetes and hyperlipidaemia, need to be addressed as medical therapy is being instituted

With the wide range of antihypertensive agents available, therapy should now be tailored to an individual case. ACE inhibitors should be used in hyper-tensive diabetics as they retard onset of microvascular complications and have a slight positive effect on lipid profiles. Doxazosin, an alpha adrenoceptor blocker, is particularly useful in resistant hypertension, where two to three agents in combination have failed to lower the blood pressure. It also has beneficial effects on the lipid profile and is therefore used in patients with associated hyperlipidaemia. In the older patient, bendrofluazide remains the first line treatment, where the lower dose of 2.5 mg once a day, (as compared to 5 mg) has been shown to be optimal.

Answer 11   Marks

(a) Phaeochromocytoma
     Cushing's syndrome
     Conn's syndrome
     Acromegaly   3

(b) Renal artery stenosis
     Polycystic kidney disease
     Renal malignant tumours   3

(c) Blood tests – FBC, U+Es, glucose, calcium / phosphate, lipids
                   autoantibody screen, ANCA, ANF

Urine –   dipstix for protein and glucose, microscopy for
          red cell casts
          consider 24-hour urine for protein and creatinine
          clearance
Imaging – plain AXR, USS of kidneys, bladder, and ureters
          consider IVU and renal DSA scan
This screen should indicate whether this is a renal or extra-renal
problem.   4

Comment
Secondary causes of hypertension are uncommon, accounting for only 5% of cases. Of these, 80% are renal or renovascular in origin and always need to be excluded in anyone presenting with hypertension. Simple bedside tests including urine dipstix and microscopy are often enough to exclude major renal disease. If there is evidence of renal dysfunction on screening, then renal imaging should be undertaken, including USS, IVP, and DSA scan. Other causes of chronic renal disease include the systemic vaculitides, which should be excluded by an autoantibody screen, in particular an ANCA test. The remaining 20% of cases are principally associated with endocrine disorders. Phaeochromocytoma, Cushing's syndrome, acromegaly, Conn's syndrome, and hyperparathyroidism may be excluded clinically, biochemically and by specific imaging and hormone assessment.

CHAPTER 7: HAEMATOLOGY ANSWERS

Answer 1   **Marks**

(a)   Iron deficiency anaemia
      Anaemia of chronic disease
      Thalassaemia trait
      Sideroblastic anaemia – primary and secondary   3

(b)   FBC, with MCV, MCH, and MCHC
      Iron studies – iron, TIBC
      Ferritin
      Haemoglobin electrophoresis – in suspected thalassaemia
      Consider bone marrow examination
      Upper and lower gastrointestinal endoscopy or barium studies
      Cervical smear and pelvic USS   3

(c)   Gastrointestinal –
            Upper: oesophagitis, oesophageal carcinoma, varices,
                    hiatus hernia,
                    peptic ulcer disease,
                    benign tumours of the stomach, e.g. leiomyoma
                    malignant tumours of the stomach
            Lower: anal fissures, haemorrhoids, rectal ulcer, rectal
                    carcinoma
                    diverticular disease, inflammatory bowel disease, colonic
                    carcinoma, infective colitis, angiodysplasia
      Extra-intestinal –
            Gynaecological:
                    fibroids, dysfunctional uterine bleeding
                    menorrhagia – primary and secondary
                    cervical and uterine carcinoma
            Epistaxis
            Urinary tract – renal tumours, polycystic kidneys
            bladder tumours   4

Comment

Anaemia is a clinical sign and wherever possible needs a definitive underlying diagnosis. Microcytic anaemia is principally caused by iron deficiency,
but may also be caused by anaemia of chronic disease, thalassaemia trait and
sideroblastic anaemia.

Iron deficiency anaemia is characterized by a hypochromic, microcytic
picture and is most commonly caused by blood loss. It is associated with a

low ferritin and low plasma iron. The commonest cause worldwide is infestation of the gut by hookworm. In the Western world, menstrual loss is the commonest cause, but in all cases gastrointestinal pathology should be excluded. Particularly in male patients over the age of 40 and postmenopausal women, malignancy must be excluded, and upper and lower gastrointestinal investigation with endoscopy or barium studies are mandatory. Anaemia of chronic disease arises secondary to chronic inflammatory disorders, such as inflammatory bowel disease, or rheumatological conditions, and is associated with a moderate reduction of the MCV, and normal iron and ferritin levels. Alpha and beta thalassaemia trait are identifiable by a disproportionate reduction in the (MCV compared to the minor level of anaemia, e.g. HB 10.5 g/dl, MCV 63 fl, (normal range 80–96 fl). They can be confirmed by haemoglobin electrophoresis. The sideroblastic anaemias are relatively uncommon. They may be congenital, due to a rare X-linked enzyme defect in the haem synthesis pathway, or acquired, secondary to malignancy, myeloproliferative disorders, and toxins, such as alcohol and lead. Often, however, no cause is found. They are characterized by ring sideroblasts in the bone marrow.

Answer 2   **Marks**

(a)   Hypothyroidism
      Pernicious anaemia/B12 deficiency   2

(b)   Pernicious anaemia is caused by one of two antibodies
      directed against intrinsic factor (IF), thus blocking B12
      absorption
      Type 1 – blocks the binding of intrinsic factor to B12
      Type 2 – blocks the IF:B12 complex binding to its receptor
      site in the terminal ileum   3

(c)   Investigations –   FBC, U+Es, TFTs, glucose
                             B12/folate
                             Autoimmune antibody screen
      Treatment –   thyroxine replacement
                             B12 injections every 3 months
      This woman should also have an upper gastrointestinal
      endoscopy to exclude carcinoma of the stomach, which
      occurs in 2% of cases   5

Comment
Macrocytosis, i.e. an MCV >96 fl, may be classified according to the presence

or absence of megaloblasts in the peripheral blood film. When associated with megaloblasts, B12 and folate deficiencies are the commonest causes. These are both classically associated with hypersegmented neutrophils. Macrocytosis in the absence of megaloblastic changes may occur physiologically in the newborn and pregnancy, and pathologically associated with chronic liver disease, alcohol abuse, hypothyroidism and reticulocytosis. Pernicious anaemia is an autoimmune disorder predominantly occurring in older women. It is commonly associated with other autoimmune disorders, including hypothyroidism, vitiligo, and Addison's disease. Auto-antibodies directed against intrinsic factor and the terminal ileal binding sites stop B12 absorption, leading to a macrocytic anaemia. Treatment of the anaemia is by intramuscular B12 injection. Initially, five 1 mg loading injections are given over two weeks, and then maintenance doses are subsequently given every three months.

Answer 3   **Marks**

(a) (i)   Alpha and beta thalassaemia
           HbSC disease
           HbD and HbE disease   2
     (ii) Acute splenic sequestration   1

(b) Treat the underlying cause of the acute sickle crisis
     IV access, IV fluids to maintain adequate hydration
     Oxygen via mask
     Appropriate analgesia – opiates
     Blood transfusion if required   3

(c) (i)   Skin – chronic leg ulceration
     (ii) Renal – acute and chronic papillary necrosis
     (iii) Biliary tree – pigmented gallstones
     (iv) Bone – aseptic necrosis of the femoral head   4

Comment
Haemolytic anaemias are characterized by features of:
- Increased red cell production (reticulocytosis)
- Increased red cell destruction (unconjugated hyperbilirubinaemia)
- Red cell damage (fragmentation and shortened red cell survival)

The haemoglobinopathies are caused by defective globin chain synthesis and all result in haemolysis of varying severity. The thalassaemias are caused by absent or abnormal production of the alpha (α) and beta (β) chains which form the normal adult haemoglobin, HbA, ($\alpha2\beta2$). The clinically significant haemoglobinopathies are summarized below.

Thalassaemia alpha

α o – homozygous – no α chain production is incompatible with life and causes the death of the foetus, termed hydrops fetalis. The resulting Hb is called Hb Barts, and has four gamma chains.

α + – heterozygotes – there is some a chain production allowing normal HbA and Hbβ4 to be produced. This gives rise to mild to moderate haemolytic disease.

Thalassaemia β

β o – homozygotes – severe haemolytic disease, requiring repeated transfusion

β + – heterozygotes – usually symptomless

$\delta\beta$ – mild to moderate disease, due to the depletion of δ chain gene. The δ chain forms part of the HbA2 which accounts for 2% of adult haemoglobin.

Sickle cell disease (HbS)

HbSS – homozygotes – this is a common haemoglobinopathy in Black races and is caused by an amino acid abnormality at position 6 of the β chain. It presents in acute sickle 'crises', usually precipitated by infection. The various organs involved are damaged through micro-infarcts, which lead to the bony pain, renal failure and chronic skin ulceration.

Heterozygotes usually remain symptomless until exposed to a stress such as hypoxia or major surgery.

HbS may combine with other Hb defects, e.g. HbS/β thalassaemia, and Hb SC disease.

The other chain defects give rise to:

- HbC disease (this is a β chain abnormality principally found in West Africa)
- HbD disease (mild haemolytic disease)
- HbE disease (this occurs mainly in South East Asia and produces a mild haemolytic disease.)

The persistence of these genetic defects is associated with protection against malarial infection.

Answer 4   **Marks**

(a)   Lymphoma – probably Hodgkin's   1

(b)   FBC and blood film, ESR
      CXR
      Lymph node biopsy
      Bone marrow trephine
      Staging CT scan of the thorax and abdomen   5

(c)   Therapeutic management depends on the stage of the disease
at presentation:-
Radiotherapy – palliative or curative
Chemotherapy – combination therapy given in cycles
Autologous bone marrow transplant – given with total body
irradiation or chemotherapy   4

Comment

Lymphomas are divided into Hodgkin's and non-Hodgkin's disease.

Hodgkin's disease has a bimodal age presentation, the early peak at 20–30 years, and the later peak over the age of 50. It is twice as common in men. The diagnosis is confirmed by histology from biopsied lymph nodes, and is characterized by the presence of the Reed–Sternberg cell. The histology also defines the classification and prognosis, as shown below.

Histological variety	Survival at 5 years (%)
Lymphocyte predominant	80–85
Nodular sclerosing	80
Mixed cellularity	60
Lymphocyte depleted	50

Each stage is subdivided into a and b, depending on the absence or presence of systemic symptoms, respectively, e.g. night sweats and pruritus.

The non-Hodgkin's lymphomas are a relatively heterogeneous group, with variable presentations and progression. They are classified by their malignant potential into low-, intermediate- and high-grade lymphomas, and by their cell type into T-cell and B-cell diseases. Certain diseases predispose to this group of malignancies, including immunosuppressive disorders, e.g. AIDS, EBV, coeliac disease, rheumatoid arthritis and SLE. The prognosis varies from 80 to 90% survival at five years in low-grade disease, to 40–50% survival in high-grade disease.

Answer 5   **Marks**

(a)   Viral respiratory tract infection, leading to immune
thrombocytopenic purpura   2

(b)   Aplastic anaemia – idiopathic (50%), drugs, sepsis
Hypersplenism, e.g. chronic haemolytic disease
Myelofibrosis
DIC
SLE   5

(c)   Usually self-limiting – can have spontaneous remissions
Steroids are used in more severe cases
In chronic disease – splenectomy or immunosuppressants   3

Comment
Reduced platelet numbers or thrombocytopenia, is characterized by purpura, easy bruising and overt bleeding, such as menorrhagia, epistaxis and gastro-intestinal bleeds. Treatment in severe cases requires blood transfusion, FFP, and platelets, although if the underlying cause is not corrected, giving platelets has little effect. In chronic thrombocytopenia treatment is principally steroids and immunosuppressants, such as azothioprine, cyclophosphamide and chlorambucil.

Thrombocytopenia may be classified into reduced platelet production or increased destruction as shown below:

* Reduced production (congenital)
* Reduced production (acquired – marrow infiltration, e.g. myelofibrosis, aplastic anaemia, drugs, e.g. omeprazole, megaloblastosis)
* Increased destruction (immune – idiopathic, viral, drugs)
* Increased destruction (microangiopathic disease – TTP, DIC, HUS)
* Increased destruction (septicaemia – usually secondary to Gram-negative organisms)

Answer 6   **Marks**

(a)   Acute lymphoblastic leukaemia (ALL)
It has a higher incidence in association with trisomy 21   2

(b)   FBC with blood film
CXR
Bone marrow aspirate and trephine
Lymph node biopsy
Chromosome analysis
Cytochemistry and immune markers   3

(c)   General supportive treatment
        – nutritional support, blood transfusions
        – neutropenic patients – isolated, infection
Prophylaxis and treatment
Specific cytotoxic therapy
Radiotherapy

Maintenance therapy
Relapse treatment – bone marrow transplant and
        chemotherapy   5

Comment

Acute lymphoblastic (ALL) and acute myeloid (AML) leukaemia present most commonly with symptoms of bone marrow failure, i.e. anaemia, recurrent infection, easy bruising and overt bleeding.

ALL presents in childhood, with bone marrow failure, hepatosplenomegaly and lymphadenopathy. Other less common sites of primary infiltration are the gums, skin, thyroid, central nervous system and testes, although these are often sites of recurrence.

The incidence of AML increases with age, and presents similarly to ALL, often with associated systemic symptoms such as malaise, fever, and lethargy. The acute leukaemias are classified by cell morphology, immunological markers and cytochemical staining. The main classification is the FAB, i.e. French, American and British.

Prognosis is now estimated at 60% at five years for ALL, but spontaneous relapses, resistance and complications to the initial treatment will significantly reduce this.

Poor prognostic indicators at presentation include:

* WCC >20
* male
* presenting age < 2 and >10 years
* B-ALL
* Philadelphia chromosome or other translocations
* central nervous system involvement
* slow remission

Answer 7   **Marks**

(a) (i) Chronic myeloid leukaemia (CML)   1
   (ii) Philadelphia chromosome. This is a reciprocal translocation
       between chromosomes 9 and 22   1

(b)   Chronic malaria
       Visceral leishmaniasis
       Myelofibrosis
       Gaucher's disease   2

(c) (i) FBC and blood film
        Chromosome analysis
        Neutrophil alkaline phosphatase score
        Bone marrow aspirate and trephine   3
    (ii) Treatment –   cytotoxic therapy
                      bone marrow transplant
                      splenic irradiation or splenectomy
                      allopurinol   3

Comment

The chronic-myeloid and lymphocytic leukaemias, (CML and CLL), present in middle and later life, although they may rarely occur in children. CML has a peak presentation between 40–60 years old, and presents with symptoms of bone marrow failure, splenomegaly, and systemic upset, such as malaise and fever. It is characterized by the presence of the Philadelphia chromosome. Treatment is aimed at producing chronic remission, but at present median survival is still only 50% at five years. Death occurs usually as the result of acute transformation, with secondary infection and severe marrow dysfunction.

CLL is usually a disorder of the elderly adult, being rare before the age of 40. It is often asymptomatic and picked up only on routine blood tests. It is classified according to the Rai staging system, as shown below:

- STAGE 0 (peripheral lymphocytosis >15 / marrow lymphocytosis >40%)
- STAGE 1 (Stage 0 + lymphadenopathy)
- STAGE 2 (Stage 1 + splenomegaly and / or hepatomegaly)
- STAGE 3 (Stage 2 + HB < 11 g/dl)
- STAGE 4 (Stage 3 + platelet count <100)

Older, asymptomatic patients often require no specific treatment, but in more advanced cases, particularly in patients with stage 3 or 4 disease, general support, i.e. nutritional and psychological support, early treatment of infection, and chemotherapy, radiotherapy and splenectomy are all employed. The median survival is 12–15 years in stage 0 disease, and 1–3 years in stage 4.

Answer 8   **Marks**

(a)   Pathological fracture
      Multiple myeloma   2

(b)   FBC and blood film
      U+Es

Calcium and phosphate
ESR
Plasma electrophoresis
Urinary Bence–Jones proteins
Bone marrow aspirate   5

(c)   IV access
       IV fluids – rehydrate using normal saline
       Principal treatment – intravenous bisphosphanates, e.g. etidronate
       consider loop diuretics, steroids, and calcitonin   3

Comment

Multiple myeloma is a malignant condition of the bone marrow, which presents after the age of 40. It is characterized by the presence of plasma cells in the marrow, lytic bone lesions, and a monoclonal paraprotein, which is found in the plasma and urine. This paraprotein is most commonly IgG, followed by IgA and IgM. IgD and combination cases are rare.

Clinically it presents with:

* Bony pain (particularly of the lower back)
* Features of bone marrow failure (anaemia, recurrent infection and overt bleeding)
* Hypercalcaemia (this produces nausea and vomiting, confusion, polyuria and polydypsia)
* Renal failure (renal impairment may be due to one of several mechanisms, deposition of light chains in the tubules, hypercalcaemia, hyperuricaemia, amyloidosis, pyelonephritis)

Treatment is based on supportive therapy and the use of alkylating agents. The use of alpha interferon post-bone marrow transplant is under investigation.

The prognosis remains relatively poor, with a median survival of 2–3 years. Poor prognostic indicators at the time of presentation include, severe anaemia, uraemia >14mmol/l, high levels of Bence–Jones proteins, raised $\beta2$-microglobulin and a low albumin.

CHAPTER 8: DERMATOLOGY ANSWERS

Answer 1 Marks

(a)   Obstructive jaundice – probably secondary to gallstones   1

(b)   Scabies
Eczema/Dermatitis
Parasitic infestation
Iron deficiency anaemia   4

(c)   Keep the patient cool
Keep skin well oiled with emollients
Avoid excessive bathing – drying
Treat the underlying disorder
Antihistamines
Sedatives
Low dose amitriptyline (nocte)
Short nails
May require occlusive bandaging of skin   5

Comment

Pruritus is a common symptom of many dermatoses and systemic disorders. The sensation is produced in the skin by various stimulants, such as brady-kinins, histamine, proteases and bile salts, and is relayed to the thalamus and sensory cortex via the lateral spinothalamic tract. There are a number of important causes of pruritus, which should always be excluded in any presentation. The commonest in the UK include insect bites and scabies, where the burrows and tracts should be sought in the skin webs of the fingers and toes. Generalized pruritus accompanies several systemic disorders. Biliary disease, particularly obstructive jaundice, present with pruritus caused by bile salt accumulation in the skin. Haematological disorders, including iron deficiency anaemia, CLL, and Hodgkins disease. Chronic uraemia classically due to PRV, chronic glomerulonephritis or chronic pyelonephritis may present with intense itching, which may be unrelieved even with dialysis. Psychological factors such as depression may decrease the threshold of pruritus. Treatment should be aimed at the underlying condition if one is readily identifiable. Symptomatic relief should include night sedation, keeping the skin well oiled with emollients, with the patient cooled. Drug therapy may include low dose amitriptyline and antihistamines. In haematological and biliary disease, a combination of H_1 and H_2 antagonists seem to produce a better response.

Answer 2   **Marks**

(a) (i) Contact dermatitis   2
     (ii) Nickel sensitivity – earrings, shampoos   1

(b) Nickel fasteners on bras
     Metal buttons on clothes, jeans, shoes
     Rubber in the elastic of underwear
     Cosmetics and perfumes   3

(c) Avoidance of sensitizers
     Should be recommended to wear gloves if continuing in her job
     Patch testing to confirm allergens
     Acute – steroid creams reduces inflammation   4

Comment

Contact dermatitis may be due to over-exposure to a particular irritant such as bleach, shampoo, cleaning agents, or may be an allergic phenomenon due to exposure to a sensitizer. Common sensitizers include cosmetics, particularly the cheaper varieties, nickel and metallic elements in clothing and shoes and plants. There are several occupation-related contact dermatoses, including hairdressers (Nickel), farmers (pesticides) and builders (chrome). Treatment is based on identification of a sensitizing allergen, and then avoidance if possible. Acutely, anti-inflammatory agents may be needed, steroid creams being most useful. Stress and the wellbeing of the patients are also very important in how the disorder is perceived and in the prognosis.

Answer 3   **Marks**

(a) Lichenification – thickening of the skin with increase of the
     skin markings due to excessive scratching and rubbing
     Flexures of the limbs and creases of the face and neck   3

(b) Atopic/extrinsic asthma   3
     Allergic rhinitis
     IgE mediated response – associated with depressed T-Cell
     response

(c) Acute treatment: Moisturization of the affected skin
                        Wet dressings with overlying dry dressing
                        Treatment of infected areas – IV antibiotics

Chapter 8: Dermatology Answers

	Avoid drying agents/irritants – soaps	
	Steroid creams	
Prevention:	Allergen avoidance – house dust mites	
	Irritant avoidance – soap, wool	
	Keep skin moisturized	
	Trial of elimination diets	
	'Short sharp bursts' of steroid creams	
	Consider Chinese herbal medicines in	
	severe cases	4

Comment

Atopic eczema is a multifactorial allergic disorder affecting the skin, with 30–50% of patients having associated atopic asthma or hayfever. Classically it presents 3–6 months post-natally, and by three years characteristically affects the flexures of the limbs and creases of the face and the neck.

The pathogenesis is based on a depressed T-cell response to environmental challenges, with an associated lack of suppression of humoral immunity, principally IgE related. The allergens involved are a heterogeneous group, including food substances, house dust mites and pollens. The skin becomes reddened, dry and intensely itchy, and subsequent scratching and rubbing leads to breaking of the epidermis, ulceration and infection. Chronically this leads to lichenification. Most patients 'grow out' of their atopy by their early teenage years, and in the absence of major irritants, their skin may return to normal. More severe cases may require systemic as well as topical steroids, and more recently, controlled studies have shown benefits of Chinese herbal remedies.

Answer 4   **Marks**

(a)   Koebner phenomenon – the rash develops in a line caused by
        the trauma of scratching
        Lichen planus; discoid lupus erythematosus; vitiligo; warts;
        eczema; secondary syphilis   3

(b)   Scalp; buttocks; truncal area
        Nails
        Joints   3

(c)   Steroids – locally – skin necrosis
        Systemically – cushingoid features
        Coal tar preparations – local irritation (rare)
        Dithranol paste – local irritation – particularly the genitalia and eyes

Phototherapy –	Psoralens – photosensitivity	
	UVA – dry/atrophy	
Systemic therapy	ACTH/steroids	
	retinoic acid – dry mouth	4

Comment

Psoriasis is a common dermatological disorder, which affects approximately 2% of the Caucasian population in the UK. It is less common in dark skinned races. It affects all age groups with a peak incidence in young adults. It is now known there are two modes of inheritance. Type I which is associated with HLA CW6, B13 and BW57 and has a strong family history. Type II is the more common and is associated with HLA CW2 and B27. Pathologically it is characterized by an increase in the rate of epidermal cell turnover. Clinically there is epidermal thickening and scaling which most commonly occur in demarcated plaques. Psoriasis may occur in several patterns:

- Guttate – this is a 'droplet' type pattern which follows a streptococcal infection. It is common in children.
- Pustular psoriasis – in this disorder pustules occur associated with a systemic upset, including pyrexia, arthropathy and erythema. It usually occurs in association with psoriatic treatment including steroids but, rarely, may be associated with hypothyroidism.
- Nummular discoid – this is the commonest form associated with well demarcated plaques over the extensor surfaces.

Answer 5   **Marks**

(a)	Erythema multiforme, Stevens–Johnson syndrome	2
(b)	Mycoplasma pneumonia	
	Herpes simplex; Streptococcus; Orf virus	
	Drugs, e.g. penicillin; sulphonamides	4

(c)	Investigations:	FBC; U+Es; LFTS
		Atypical pneumonia screen; Mycoplasma;
		Legionella; Chlamydia
		CXR; ABGs
	Treatment:	Treat the underlying cause – amoxycillin
		and erythromycin
		Systemic steroids
		Nutrition must be addressed if prolonged
		mouth ulceration stops oral intake

The marks for section (c) total 4.

Chapter 8: Dermatology Answers

Comment

Erythema multiforme is characterized by the target lesion, which is a red annular lesion with a blistering centre. The rash predominantly affects the peripheries, but may also involve the trunk, genitalia, eyes and mouth. Common causes include:

- Bacteria (streptococcus, mycoplasma)
- Viruses (HSV, Orf)
- Fungi (histoplasmosis, coccidioidomycosis)
- Drugs (penicillins, sulphonamides, NSAIDs)
- Inflammatory bowel disease
- Rheumatoid arthritis and SLE
- Neoplasia
- DXT and CXT

The Stevens–Johnson syndrome is a severe form of the more common erythema multiforme, presenting with blistering and mucosal involvement. It may be associated with multi-organ failure, and requires immediate attention. Treatment is based on symptomatic relief and treatment of the underlying disorder. The more severe Stevens–Johnson syndrome requires systemic steroids.

Answer 6	**Marks**

(a) Erythema nodosum — 1

(b) Infection – TB
Drugs – Sulphonamides
IBD
Sarcoidosis — 4

(c) Stop oral contraceptive pill (OCP); use other forms of contraception
Analgesia with aspirin; bedrest
Treat underlying infection if present
Steroids – if not settling — 5

Comment

Erythema nodosum is characterized by painful, tender red lesions, which are often ill-defined, and merge into one another. They occur over the anterior aspect of the shins, the forearms and more rarely the truncal area. Common causes include:

- Infection (Bacterial – streptococcal, TB, LGV, leprosy; Viral – EBV;

Fungal – histoplasmosis, blastomycosis, coccidioidomycosis)
- Sarcoidosis
- IBD
- Drugs (sulphonamides, OCP, bromides)
- Pregnancy
- Malignancy (leukaemia, lymphoma)

Management is based on treating the underlying cause. A chest X-ray is mandatory as sarcoidosis and tuberculosis are common associations. The rash is self-limiting but aspirin and bedrest are recommended. Steroids may help with swelling and fever, but do not change the duration of the illness. They may also be indicated for treatment of the underlying disorder.

Answer 7 **Marks**

(a) Pemphigus vulgaris; pemphigoid; fixed drug eruption;
     insect bites   3

(b) Do you have any ulcers/blisters in the mouth?
     Have you started any new medications recently?
     Have you been in contact with any biting insects recently,
     e.g. mites or mosquitos?   3

(c) (i) Nikolsky's sign – sliding pressure applied to the
          edge of a lesion will cause the epidermis to break away
          Pemphigus vulgaris   2
     (ii) Steroids – mainstay of therapy
          Immunosuppressants – azathioprine; cyclophosphamide 2

Comment

Pemphigus is an autoimmune disorder caused by an antibody to epidermal intracellular components. It is associated with HLA-A10 and DR4, and is more common in Jews and in the Indian subcontinent. Clinically it presents with superficial blistering/erosive lesions, with a predilection to the buccal mucosa. The lesions classically exhibit Nikolsky's sign. Treatment is based on high dose oral or IV steroids, with immunosuppressants now used as steroid saving agents. Most patients are cured and therapy is usually stopped within two years.

Pemphigoid is a more common disorder than pemphigus, and presents with large, tense, bullous eruptions, principally in the over 60s population. It is unusual for it to affect the mouth. It is also an immune mediated disorder and in 70% of cases there is a specific IgG targeted against the basement membrane of the epidermis. The treatment is similar to pemphigus, with most patients cured within one year.

Answer 8   **Marks**

(a)   Rapid increasing size
       Itching
       Bleeding – spontaneous
       Irregular margins
       Development of any new pigmented lesion after puberty
       Associated surrounding lesions
       Distant similar lesions
       Recent change in surface
       Change in colour
       Lymph node enlargement   4

(b)   BCC; SCC; solar keratoses; malignant melanoma; Bowens
       disease   3

(c)   Excision of naevus
       Chemotherapy for metastatic disease
       Advice about sunlight avoidance   3

Comment
The incidence of malignant melanoma is rapidly increasing within Caucasian populations, particularly in the UK. This is thought to be principally due to Celtic, 'red haired' races, subjecting themselves to short sharp bursts of intense sunbathing on summer holidays. The most important prognostic indicator is the depth of the lesion:
*   <0.76 mm   (95% survival/5 years)
*   >0.76–1 mm (80% survival/5 years)
*   >3.5 mm   (40% survival/5 years)
Recent studies have shown that wide excision with regional lymph node dissection has no advantage over less radical surgery, and presently the recommendation is 1 cm excision margins for every 1 mm in depth. Trials continue with various forms of chemotherapy, including interferon, retinoids and other agents, but as yet none have been shown to greatly influence prognosis.
Prophylaxis with ongoing education about the importance of 'covering up' in the sun, and the use of sun-screening agents, has been shown to be a successful influence in Australasia and southern Africa.

Chapter 8: Dermatology Answers

Answer 9   **Marks**

(a)   Thyrotoxicosis
       Psoriasis   2

(b)   TFTs
       Nail clippings/scraping – UV (Wood's light)
       Thyroid auto-antibodies
       HLA (B27) – Karyotyping   2

(c)   i)   Koilonychia
       ii)   Clubbing
       iii)   Splinter haemorrhages and clubbing
       iv)   Pitting; transverse ridging; dystrophy; onycholysis
       v)   Beau's lines
       vi)   Leukonychia; clubbing   6

Comment

The nails of the digits continue to grow throughout life. Retardation in growth may occur in severe psychiatric or systemic disease, acceleration of nail growth, principally occurring in psoriasis.

The shape of the nails vary in numerous systemic disorders.

Clubbing of the nail

Classically this is an increase in the curvature of the nail in both longitudinal and transverse planes, with loss of the angle between the nail bed and skin fold. The nail bed becomes fluctuant. Causes include:

- Idiopathic
- Chronic suppurative lung disease (CF, bronchiectasis, empyema, TB, abscess)
- Pulmonary malignancy
- Congenital cyanotic heart disease
- Infective endocarditis
- Inflammatory bowel disease
- Chronic liver disease
- Biliary disease

Onycholysis

This is separation of the distal portion of the nail, causing it to appear white. It arises due to trauma or association with psoriasis and thyrotoxicosis.

Beau's Lines

These are transverse white lines due to psychiatric or systemic disease, which cause a temporary cessation of growth. They also occur when chemotherapy is used.

Pitting

Arises due to localized increase in nail growth, classically seen in psoriasis. Pitting may also occur in eczema.

Answer 10   **Marks**

(a)   Older sister – alopecia areata   1
        Younger sister – hirsutism   1

(b)   Older: autoimmune disease – pernicious anaemia; Addison's
                disease; atopy; familial
        Younger: racial; polycystic ovaries syndrome; congenital
                adrenal hyperplasia; drugs; puberty; adrenal carcinoma;
                menopause   4

(c)   i)   Racial/simple hirsutism – cosmetic advice – depilation
                creams; electrolysis; bleaching
        ii)   Polycystic ovary syndrome – anti-androgens –
                Cyproterone or dionette   4

Comment

Loss of hair in well defined areas is termed alopecia areata. It is an immune mediated disorder with CD4 T-cell infiltration of the hair bulb. It may be familial, and there is often a strong history of atopy. It has an association with autoimmune diseases, including thyrotoxicosis, and hypothyroidism; PA, Addison's disease and vitiligo, and it is also seen in Down's syndrome. Most cases will respond to treatment of the underlying disease and spontaneously resolve. Intradermal steroids in affected areas encourages hair re-growth but may also cause atrophy of the overlying skin, and thus cause re-loss in several months. Hirsutism is the term given to growth of hair in the male distribution. Hypertrichosis is the term given to growth of hair in 'ectopic' sites not normally associated with hair growth. Hirsutism may be racial, physiological, e.g. puberty and post-menopausal, and pathological due to endocrine disorders. Amenorrhoea and menstrual irregularity, acne, obesity and poor breast development should alert the doctor to more sinister pathology. Examination should exclude signs of virilization including clitoromegaly. The principal pathologies associated with these signs are polycystic ovaries; congenital adrenal hyperplasia; virilizing tumours of the adrenals and ovaries and Cushing's disease.

Chapter 8: Dermatology Answers

Answer 11   **Marks**

(a)   Albinism
      Tuberculoid leprosy
      Pityriasis versicolor (dark skinned patients)   3

(b)   Diabetes mellitus
      Addison's disease
      Pernicious anaemia
      Thyroid disease – thyrotoxicosis and myxoedema   3

(c)   FBC – including MCV; U+E;
      B12 and folate
      Glucose
      Auto antibody screen – IF, thyroid   4

Comment

Vitiligo is a commonest cause of depigmentation its incidence varying from 1% in the UK to almost 9% in the Indian sub-continent. It is an autoimmune disorder, but the triggering factors have not as yet been identified. A family history is positive in 33% of cases. Common associations include pernicious anaemia, Addison's disease, thyrotoxicosis, myxoedema and diabetes. On presentation, evidence of other autoimmune disease should always be sought. The lesions of vitiligo are usually symmetrical, and in 50% of cases are apparent before the age of 20 years. They may occur in sites of trauma, such as the knuckles or around a naevus, known as a halo naevus. They may also exhibit the Koebner phenomenon. Other causes of depigmentation include:

• Albinism (partial or complete)
• Phenylketonuria
• Tuberculoid leprosy (associated with anaesthesia)
• Pityriasis versicolor caused by *Malassezia furfur*
• Syphilis
• Ash leaf spots of Tuberose sclerosis
• Post-inflammatory depigmentation = *Pityriasis alba* (this occurs in psoriasis and eczema)

CHAPTER 9: GASTROENTEROLOGY ANSWERS

Answer 1   **Marks**

(a)   Clinical features:
        No impact pain on swallowing, weight loss or cachexia
        No cervical adenopathy or anaemia
        Investigations:
        Barium swallow and/or
        Oesophagoscopy and mucosal biopsy   3

(b)   (i)   By oesophageal manometry: a pressure transducer
                on a lead is swallowed and records the intra-luminal
                and sphincter pressures during swallowing
                By video fluoroscopy of swallow   2
        (ii)   Achalasia of the cardia (cardiospasm)
                Degenerative changes in vagal innervation and
                muscular hypertrophy of the lower third of the
                oesophagus producing a functional obstruction   2

(c)   Forceful dilatation of the lower oesophageal sphincter with a
        hydrostatic balloon under imaging. Failure of repeated dilatations
        is an indication for cardiomyotomy (Heller's operation)   3

Comment
In patients with dysphagia, a malignant lesion must be excluded as a first step.
Inflammatory strictures due to acid reflux from hiatus hernia and accidental
ingestion of corrosives in children are more frequently encountered. Myas-
thaenia gravis or motor neurone disease may present with dysphagia due to a
defect in neuromuscular transmission. Other causes are progressive systemic
sclerosis, some connective tissue disorders and Chagas' disease (American
trypanasomiasis). Oesophageal candidiasis, which is readily diagnosed on
endoscopy, is frequently regarded as an AIDS-defining illness and an
indication for immunological screening.

Answer 2   **Marks**

(a)   Hiatus hernia with reflux oesophagitis
        The lower oesophageal sphincter and the sphincter mechanism
        of the crura of the diaphragm are incompetent, resulting in
        equalization of intra-gastric and oesophageal pressures,
        producing reflux of stomach and duodenal contents into the
        oesophagus   3

243

(b)   Oesophageal pH monitoring: a pH probe is placed in the
       distal oesophagus and acid exposure is monitored in the
       ambulatory state and at rest. The patient's symptoms are
       correlated with the actual recording of acid reflux episodes.
       Acid perfusion (Bernstein) test: Symptoms of acid reflux
       may be reproduced by dripping dilute acid via a nasogastric
       tube into the distal oesophagus   3

(c)   General measures: liquid or chewable antacids (aluminium or
       magnesium hydroxide 30 ml 30 min after meals and at bed
       time). Alginic acid antacids (Gaviscon 10 ml 30 min after
       meals and at bed time).
       Elevate head of bed on blocks. Avoid alcohol, smoking, fatty
       and spicy food, and food or drink before bed time. Lose weight.
       Specific measures for severe symptoms:
       Promotility drugs: bethanechol 10–15 mg qid, metoclopromide
       10 mg qid
       H$_2$ receptor blockers: cimetidine 400 mg bid, ranitidine
       150 mg bid
       In the presence of severe oesophagitis, omeprazole,
       Lansoprazole or pantoprazole 20 mg is added to the above.
       Anti-reflux surgery (fundoplication) should be considered in
       severe, intractable cases   4

Comment

Gastro-oesophageal reflux disease is usually associated with a sliding hernia,
which interferes with normal oesophageal clearance by acting as a fluid trap.
Endoscopic changes in the lower oesophagus range from shallow linear
erosions to confluent ulcers to complete mucosal destruction (Grades I to IV).
Metaplastic changes to columnar epithelium of the lower oesophagus
(Barrett's oesophagus) is produced by severe chronic reflux and is associated
with the development of an adenocarcinoma.

Answer 3   **Marks**

(a)   Peptic ulcer disease   2

(b)   OGD or barium meal examination
       Visualization or imaging of the ulcer in the stomach or
       duodenum, with associated deformity or scarring of the
       pyloro-duodenum. The amount of gastric residue and the

volume of the stomach may suggest delayed gastric emptying
due to pyloric stenosis caused by the ulcer   3

(c)   In symptomatic disease, where there is no evidence of *H. pylori*
        infection, the patients should be given *one* of the following:
        Cimetidine 400 mg BD and 800 mg nocte for 2–3 months
        Ranitidine 150 mg BD and 300 mg nocte for 2–3 months
        Omeprazole 20 mg daily for 4 weeks
        Lansoprazole 30 mg daily for 4 weeks

        Where there is evidence of *H. pylori* infection, triple therapy
        should be given for <u>ONE</u> week only:

        Lansoprazole 30 mg BD   or   Omeprazole 20 mg BD
        Clarithromycin 500 mg BD   Clarithromycin 500 mg BD
        Amoxycillin 1 g BD   or
                                         Amoxycillin 1 g BD
                                         and
                                         Metronidazole 400 mg BD
                                                                        5

        Treatment with a proton pump inhibitor or H_2 antagonist may be
        continued for 1–2 months after completion of triple therapy to
        promote ulcer healing.

Comment
General lifestyle measures to promote ulcer healing and to prevent recurrences
would include stopping smoking and alcohol consumption, regular meals and
sufficient rest. The avoidance of aspirin and non-steroidal anti-inflammatory
agents is desirable. In addition to a healthier life style, acid secretion may be
reduced, particularly at night, by long-term maintenance therapy with H_2-
receptor blockers. Over 80% of duodenal ulcers heal with a two-month course.
Thereafter, patients may continue on a low-dose maintenance therapy aimed at
reducing nocturnal acid secretion or may take the tablets if and when
symptoms recur. A significant underlying factor in peptic ulcer disease is
Helicobacter pylori infection which is associated with 90–95% of duodenal
ulcers. This is diagnosed by bacteriological and histological examination of
antral biopsies obtained during OGD.

Answer 4   **Marks**

(a)   (i)   Malabsorption and steatorrhoea are found in:
                Blind loop syndrome with bacterial overgrowth

		Coeliac disease	
		Pancreatic enzyme deficiency	
		Bile salt deficiency	
		Tropical sprue	3
	(ii)	Duodenal biopsy showing	
		Mucosal flattening; total/partial villous atrophy	
		or raised anti-endomesial antibody titres	2
(b)	(i)	Coeliac disease (gluten-induced enteropathy)	2
	(ii)	Small bowel lymphoma/carcinoma	
		Dermatitis herpetiformis	3

Comment

Steatorrhoea implies malabsorption of fat, with faecal fat excretion in excess of 6 g/day, and signifies an inability to absorb a significant amount of the dietary constituents. The diagnosis in this patient involves distinguishing between an enteropathy and other causes of steatorrhoea. In coeliac disease there is mucosal sensitivity to wheatgerm, barley, rye and, occasionally, oats. The resulting malabsorption involves not only fat and fat soluble vitamins but also minerals and water soluble vitamins. Other causes of malabsorption are obstructive jaundice, pancreatitis, inflammatory bowel disease and overgrowth of bowel organisms.

Treatment is aimed at the cause. In obstructive jaundice bile flow is surgically re-established; pancreatic exocrine insufficiency is treated with pancreatic extract. Acute exacerbations of Crohn's disease and ulcerative colitis is treated with aminosalicylates or sulphasalazine with the addition of immuno-suppression (azathioprine) and steroids (prednisolone). Bacterial overgrowth in bowel is encountered in severe malnutrition and is treated with antibiotics and an initial elemental diet.

Answer 5   Marks

(a)		Ulcerative colitis	
		Crohn's disease	
		Infective colitis (campylobacter/amoebic colitis,	
		bacillary dysentery, pseudomembranous colitis)	
		Ischaemic colitis	
		Diverticulitis	3
(b)	(i)	Acute ulcerative colitis	1
	(ii)	Perforation	

Haemorrhage
Toxic megacolon   3

(c)   Bed rest with close monitoring of clinical parameters
Nasogastric aspiration
IV rehydration
IV steroids (+/– azathioprine)
IV antibiotics
Blood transfusion (if anaemic)
Surgery for progressive toxicity, severe haemorrhage or
toxic megacolon   3

Comment
The diagnosis of inflammatory bowel disease is usually obvious from a history
of relapses and remissions, with progressive deterioration in symptoms,
culminating in an acute episode. In ulcerative colitis the rectal mucosa is
usually involved, with a variable proximal colonic extension, whilst Crohn's
disease mainly involves the distal small bowel, with occasional colonic
involvement. However, in 10% of cases of colitis a definitive diagnosis of
either ulcerative colitis or Crohn's disease is not possible. Inflammatory bowel
disease is treated by oral aminosalicylates or sulphasalazine. During acute
exacerbations intravenous steroids (hydrocortisone) are administered with
antibiotics when the risks of complications are high in severe disease. However,
for the vast majority of sufferers dietary measures alone or with a maintenance
dose of aminosalicylates is sufficient to keep the disease in remission.
Toxic megacolon in ulcerative colitis requires emergency colectomy.

Answer 6   **Marks**

(a)   (i)   Diarrhoea, abdominal pain, weight loss, fever,
malaise, lethargy, anorexia, nausea, vomiting   2
(ii)   Biliary: pericholangitis (19%), calculi
Kidney: oxalate stone (30%)
Joints: sacroilitis (15–18%),
monoarticular arthritis (14%)
Eye: uveitis (4%)
Skin: erythema nodosum; pyoderma gangrenosum   2

(b)   IV rehydration and electrolyte correction
IV or oral corticosteroid therapy to control the
inflammatory exacerbation

Oral aminosalicylates or sulphasalazine for
induction and maintenance of remission
Oral immunosuppression (azathioprine) to maintain
steroid-induced remission
Oral or IV antibiotic therapy (metronidazole with a
cephalosporin or cotrimoxazole) to counter bacterial
infection
Bowel rest with total parenteral nutrition or elemental diet
Correct anaemia if present   3

(c)   Surgery is reserved for complications of the disease:
bowel stenosis, fistulation or perforation, abscess
formation and rarely haemorrhage. 80% of patients
may require bowel resection at some stage of their
disease.   3

Comment

Crohn's disease is a chronic mucosal inflammation of uncertain aetiology affecting any part of the gastrointestinal tract. Characteristic microvascular abnormalities have been demonstrated in the lamina propria. Focal arteritis and arterial occlusion leads to haemorrhage and tissue ischaemia with new vessel formation which is thought to be initiated by cytokines and angiogenesis tissue factors. The disease may be confined to one segment of bowel, manifest as multiple skip lesions or involve the entire small and/or large bowel. The affected bowel is thickened and narrowed, with ulceration and fissuring of the mucosa. There may be associated fistulae and abscess formation. These, along with significant bowel stenosis, require surgical measures to eradicate infection or to restore bowel continuity. The long-term risk of bowel cancer is negligible in Crohn's disease, unlike ulcerative colitis.

Answer 7   **Marks**

(a)   (i)   B-cell lymphoma of the bowel
              Lymphoid hyperplasia of the bowel
              Kaposi's sarcoma of the bowel   2
       (ii)   Cytomegalovirus
              Microsporidium or cryptosporidium parvum
              Mycobacterium avium intercellulare   3

(b)   (i)   Plain abdominal X-ray
              CT scan of abdomen

Barium enema (for large bowel obstruction)   2
  (ii) 'Drip and suck' regime to reduce bowel activity and
       allow the lymphoidal enlargement causing the
       obstruction to regress
       The presence of an intussusception causing acute
       obstruction requires early surgical relief   3

Comment

Due to their suppressed immunity, patients with AIDS are prone to recurrent bowel infections from a wide variety of pathogens. Treatment of the atypical bowel infections with antibiotics is prolonged, and these patients are susceptible to recurrent infections. Acute or chronic intussusception may be produced by lymphatic hyperplasia or a lymphoma. The diagnosis is often delayed due to the non-specific nature of the symptoms and to the extensive differential diagnosis of abdominal pathology in these patients. The early use of CT in diagnosing bowel obstruction should forestall complications of bowel ischaemia and peritonitis.

Answer 8   **Marks**

(a) (i) Contact bleeding with mucosal friability
        Mucosal ulceration
        Mucosal granuloma (amoeboma)   3
   (ii) Serology: amoebic fluorescent antibody titres and
        precipitating antibody titres may be elevated
        Microscopy: examination of wet smears of colonic scrapings
        for cysts and trophozoites   2

(b)   Abnormal liver function tests, viz raised serum alkaline
       phosphatase
       Liver imaging by ultrasound or radionuclide scan   2

(c)   Metronidazole or tinidazole
       Dihydroemetine or chloroquine
       Diloxanide furoate (furamide)   3

Comment

Amoebiasis is common in the tropics and is an important cause of imported fever in Britain. It is transmitted in the encysted form via the oro-faecal route and produces a chronic infection of the large bowel. Pain in the right iliac fossa may simulate acute appendicitis, or chronic diarrhoea, and passage of blood-stained mucus may simulate ulcerative colitis. Granuloma formation may be palpable in the rectum or produce a filling defect in the colon on barium enema and must be distinguished from a carcinoma. Hepatic amoebiasis may present without a history of bowel symptoms. A swinging pyrexia and an enlarged, tender liver with shoulder-tip pain are characteristic of abscess formation. The latter responds well to chemotherapy but may require repeated ultrasound guided aspiration to aid resolution.

Answer 9   **Marks**

(a) (i)   Chronic pancreatitis   1
     (ii) Moderate elevation of serum amylase titres   1

(b)   Destruction of the exocrine pancreatic tissue leads to
           a fall in digestive enzyme secretion resulting in
           malabsorption. Progressive destruction of the Islet
           cells of the pancreas leads to diabetes mellitus   3

(c)   Exocrine enzyme insufficiency is treated by oral
           pancreatic enzyme supplements, the dose of which is
           titrated to reduce steatorrhoea and bowel frequency. A
           neutral duodenal pH to optimise the effect of the
           supplements is achieved by antacids or H_2 receptor
           blockers in those that respond poorly
           Endocrine (insulin) insufficiency is treated by soluble
           insulin, as oral hypoglycaemic agents are usually
           ineffective
           General measures include alcohol rehabilitation,
           supervision of analgesic use and diet   5

Comment
A nutritious and balanced diet, with fat-soluble vitamins (suitably adjusted for diabetics), with abstinence from alcohol, are the mainstay of treatment. Pancreatic pain is difficult to treat; whilst abstinence is essential to reduce the frequency and severity of attacks, analgesics, frequently narcotic agents, may have to be resorted to for pain relief. Percutaneous nerve block (coeliac plexus block) with phenol may be tried if the above measures fail. Over a 10-year period, about one-third of patients obtain relief of pain without surgical treatment, and the pain is reduced in a further one-third. The remainder have progressive symptoms, with a 50% survival over this period. Surgery in this group takes the form of internal pancreatic duct drainage or pancreatic resection, but is of little value in the patient who cannot abstain from alcohol.

Chapter 9: Gastroenterology Answers

Answer 10   **Marks**

(a)   Yellow discolouration of abdominal skin
      Ascites
      Splenomegaly
      Spider naevi
      Caput medusae
      Skin bruising
      Purpuric rash
      Skin pigmentation   3

(b)   Raised plasma bilirubin: unconjugated fraction signifies
      extent of liver damage
      Low total plasma proteins and albumin: diminished liver
      synthesis
      Raised alanine and aspartate amino-transferases: both raised
      in liver disease; alanine transferase more specific in liver
      damage
      Raised gamma-glutamyl transferase: specific for liver
      damage; distinguishes from bone disease
      Raised plasma globulin fraction: indicates underlying liver
      inflammation, e.g. hepatitis B infection
      Raised alkaline phosphatase: non-specific for liver disease
      Raised urinary bilirubin: indicates cholestasis due to hepatic
      inflammation   4

(c)   Gastrointestinal haemorrhage as a result of chronic liver
      disease (cirrhosis) is due to:
      portal hypertension leading to gastro-oesophageal varices
      increased incidence of peptic ulceration
      coagulopathy   3

Comment
The main objectives of treating patients with cirrhosis are to ensure good
nutritional status, manage chronic cholestasis and treat complications such as
ascites, portal hypertension, hepatic encephalopathy, renal failure and infection. The prognosis in cirrhosis is dependent on the extent of liver damage as
reflected by liver function. There is a 50% five-year survival when the patient
presents early with satisfactory liver compensation. The prognosis is
favourable where the cause is correctable, as in alcoholism, haemachroma-
tosis and Wilson's disease.

251

Answer 11   **Marks**

(a)   The clinical spectrum ranges from non-specific symptoms
      without detectable abnormality to acute liver failure or
      advanced cirrhosis
      Alcoholic hepatitis may be a severe illness, with a tender
      hepatomegaly and cholestatic jaundice
      It may resolve completely if the insult is removed and no
      lasting liver damage is present
      Irreversible liver damage leads to cirrhosis, which may
      present as portal hypertension, ascites or encephalopathy,
      characterizing end-stage liver disease   4

(b)   Early liver lesion: fatty change/infiltration (reversible)
      Alcoholic hepatitis: inflammatory cell infiltration with foci
      of hepatocyte necrosis
      Mallory's hyaline: pink-staining inclusion bodies found in
      inflamed hepatocytes
      Central hyaline sclerosis: fibrosis around central veins
      Cirrhosis: initially micro-nodular progressing to macro-nodular
      cirrhosis
      Mild siderosis: iron deposits in hepatocytes   3

(c)   Abstinence from alcohol is an important prognostic factor
      as it promotes complete resolution of fatty change, halts the
      progressive necrosis of hepatocytes, and improves health and
      survival
      Progressive alcoholic hepatitis results in a significant
      mortality from acute liver failure; those who recover may
      progress to cirrhosis, in which hepatocyte destruction and
      fibrosis of the liver produce end-stage liver disease
      Variceal bleeding, ascites, encephalopathy and hepato-cellular
      carcinoma are grave complications of alcoholic cirrhosis   3

Comment
Alcoholic liver disease is common in many societies, and the extent and
severity of the liver damage caused is directly related to the duration of alcohol abuse and the amount consumed daily. It is frequently difficult to obtain a
history of excessive drinking from the patient and it is useful to question the
relatives. Peripheral macrocytosis and a raised gamma-glutamyl transferase
suggest the diagnosis. Definitive treatment of irreversible alcoholic liver

damage is by liver transplantation, and in order to make this treatment cost-effective, complete abstinence must be demonstrated by the patient.

Answer 12   **Marks**

(a)   Parenteral via peripheral or central venous access
       Enteral, i.e. via the gut   2

(b)   BMI = <u>weight in kilogrammes</u>
              (height in metres)^2

       FBC, U&Es, glucose, albumin, calcium, magnesium
       Trace elements, e.g. zinc
       Ferretin, B12 and folate   4

(c)   Is the gut working? Severe gut dysmotility is a contra-
       indication to the use of enteral feeding, e.g. paralytic ileus
       Catabolic states, e.g. sepsis, burns – requires increased
       nitrogen load
       Renal impairment – limit protein (nitrogen) content and
       volume of the feed
       Liver failure – limit protein content
       Diabetes mellitus – limit carbohydrate content and
       requires insulin cover
       Duration of morbidity – if prolonged requires long-term
       enteral feeding   4

Comment

On admission to hospital all patients should have a simple nutritional assessment. The patient's present weight and height should be recorded and their 'usual' weight (and when last weighed) should also be ascertained. Any patient who has, by these simple criteria, lost 10% of their 'usual' weight is in need of nutritional support. In deciding what form of nutritional help they require, one simple rule must be followed: 'If the gut is working, use it'. If the patient is relatively well and is able to eat and drink, build-up drinks should be used. These contain approximately 500 kilocalories, essential vitamins and trace elements. They are most often used to supplement an inadequate diet. In more severe cases, such as dysphagia secondary to CVA, bulbar palsy, or motor neurone disease, gastrostomy or jejunostomy feeding is used. This is also the first line choice of patients who require long-term feeding. When the bowel is dysfunctional, e.g. mechanical obstruction, high output diarrhoea or in short bowel syndrome, parenteral feeding is indicated. Peripheral venous feeding is used to supplement the diet for short periods of time. It is limited due to the phlebitic nature of certain elements of the feeds. In prolonged and debilitating illness, feeding is through tunnelled central venous lines and the nutritional contents tailored to the individual needs.

Answer 13   **Marks**

(a)   Oesophageal varices   1
       Oesophagitis, Mallory–Weiss tear, gastritis, peptic ulcer
       disease   2

(b)   FBC, U&Es, glucose, LFTs, clotting screen, cross-match (at
       least six units)   3

(c)   Lie patient head down (in left lateral position if vomiting)
       Intravenous access – one large bore venflon in either forearm
       If any signs of shock insert central venous line
       Start colloid infusion or, if severe bleed, start blood transfusion
       with Rhesus O negative blood
       Start blood transfusion with cross-matched blood, FFP and
       platelets transfusion as required
       Give IV vitamin K if deranged INR
       Arrange upper GI endoscopy and urgent surgical assessment
       If ongoing variceal bleeding consider insertion of
       Sengstaken–Blakemore tube   4

Comment

The prognosis in acute upper GI bleeds has not changed since the 1960s despite the advent of endoscopy and earlier surgical intervention. Overall mortality is 8–12% but in specialist units it can be as low as 4%. Mortality increases with age, to over 50% in the over 75-year-olds. (The ageing population is thought to be one of the reasons for the lack of prognostic improvement.) The principal prognostic indicator in this group is re-bleeding. In patients with concurrent peptic ulcer disease, the endoscopic appearances of fresh blood clot or visible vessels in the ulcer crater both signify a high risk. Identifying these patients and treating them aggressively improves their prognosis. Oesophageal varices arise due to portal hypertension from chronic liver disease. Variceal bleeds tend to be torrential and are exacerbated by coagulopathy secondary to loss of vitamin K dependent factors and thrombocytopaenia. These carry a poor prognosis, with 50% of patients dying within six weeks of their first bleed. Therapy should be based on initial resuscitation, endoscopy and injection of sclerosant or banding of the varices. If the bleeding is difficult to stem, a continuous intravenous infusion of vasopressin should be used to reduce the portal blood flow. Vasopressin is a powerful vasoconstrictor, which constricts the splanchnic circulation and thus reduces venous pressure. Unfortunately it also causes coronary vasoconstriction and may cause cardiac ischaemia. Systemic side effects are avoided by giving a synchronous GTN infusion or the vasopressin analogue, terlipressin. The somatostatin analogue, octreotide, is also used. Transjugular intrahepatic portal systemic shunt (TIPSS) may be used for torrential variceal bleeds. This is a stented shunt between the portal and hepatic veins, which leads to decompression of the portal system.

Answer 14   **Marks**

(a)   Dyspeptic history or ingestion of alcohol, steroids and non-
          steroid anti-inflammatory agents are linked to peptic ulcer disease
          A violent bout of vomiting or retching is linked to an oesophageal
          mucosal tear
          Anorexia, weight loss, malaise may be associated with
          gastric cancer
          History of liver disease is linked to variceal haemorrhage   4

(b)   OGD   2

(c)   Endoscopic biopsies for histological confirmation
          FBC: for anaemia
          LFTs: to assess liver function
          U&Es: to assess renal function
          Liver imaging for metastatic tumour deposits
          Definitive treatment: a form of gastrectomy or a by-pass if
          unresectable with/without radiotherapy/chemotherapy   4

Comment

In the presence of hypovolaemia, CVP monitoring along with a blood transfusion is mandatory. Peptic ulcer bleeds may be controlled by submucous adrenaline injection or laser photocoagulation. Omeprazole is more effective in preventing re-bleeds than H_2 receptor blockers. In variceal haemorrhage, vasopressin or octreotide, which reduce splanchnic blood flow, along with proton pump inhibition, may be effective before proceeding to interventional procedures. Surgical resection is the only cure for gastric cancer. Palliation for advanced disease is unfortunately poor.

CHAPTER 10: NEPHROLOGY ANSWERS

Answer 1   **Marks**

(a)   Acute left-sided pyelonephritis   1

(b)   FBC, U+Es, glucose
       Blood cultures
       MSU; urinalysis
       Plain AXR   4

(c)   Immediate management –
          IV access
          IV fluids
          antiemetics and analgesia
          IV broad spectrum antibiotics – gentamicin and
          cefuroxime
       Secondary investigation –
          USS of kidneys, ureter and bladder
          IVU
          consider micturating cystogram to exclude
          vesicoureteric reflux   5

Comment

Pyelonephritis is an infective condition of the kidney, that may present in an acute or chronic manner. In the acute form, the patient presents with loin pain, fever, rigors, and nausea and vomiting. Severe cases with bilateral renal involvement may present with acute renal failure. Treatment should include symptom relief and intravenous antibiotics, particularly gentamicin.

Chronic pyelonephritis, has recently been retermed 'reflux nephropathy', as it is principally caused by chronic vesicoureteric reflux. This condition arises due to abnormalities of the ureters, which in turn lead to retrograde urinary regurgitation through the vesicoureteric junction. The kidneys therefore become scarred, atrophic and on imaging are small and have classically blunted calyces. The diagnosis may be made coincidentally on routine abdominal ultrasound scan, as it is often asymptomatic for many years. Classically it presents in childhood with recurrent urinary tract infections and loin pain. Other presenting features are renal failure, persistent proteinuria, hypertension, and renal calculi.

Treatment of vesicoureteric reflux largely depends on the stage of the disease at presentation. In children that present early with moderate to severe disease, there is a place for corrective surgery. In later presentations, or in mild to moderate disease there is little evidence to suggest that surgery changes overall outcome, and these patients should be managed conservatively, with careful monitoring of their renal function and low dose prophylactic antibiotics.

Answer 2   **Marks**

(a)   Bilateral hydronephrosis
       Bilateral renal tumours, e.g. renal carcinoma   2

(b)   Haematuria – associated with bleeding into cysts, recurrent
       UTIs, and more rarely renal carcinoma
       Recurrent UTIs
       Loin pain – this may be due to infection, bleeding into cysts
       and to the renal enlargement, which causes a non-specific,
       dull loin pain
       Hypertension
       Chronic renal failure
       Renal carcinoma – this is a rare complication   5

(c)   Treat hypertension and UTIs
       Regular follow up in renal outpatients to monitor renal function
       In end stage disease they require dialysis and renal transplantation
       Genetic counselling for patient and family   3

Comment
Polycystic kidney disease is the commonest inherited disorder to affect the kidney, and is responsible for 8–10% of end stage renal failure seen in the UK. It has two modes of inheritence, autosomal dominant, classically termed adult polycystic kidney disease, and infantile disease, which is an autosomal recessive disorder. The abnormal gene locus (PKD1), responsible for the majority of the adult cases, has been localized to the short arm of chromosome 16, another locus (PKD2), has been isolated to chromosome 4.
Both disorders are associated with cystic disease in several other intra-abdominal organs, including the liver, pancreas, spleen and ovaries (this should not be confused with polycystic ovary syndrome). The infantile form is also associated with hepatic fibrosis and portal hypertension.
Although it is occassionally discovered in childhood, the adult form usually presents in the 3rd to 4th decades, with local and systemic complications. Systemic complications and associations include:
•   Hypertension (it is important to control hypertension as this accelerates renal failure)

- Polycythaemia (due to increased erythropoetin secretion)
- Liver cysts (these occur in 70% of patients)
- Berry aneurysms (patients present with subarachnoid haemorrhage. All patients should be asked about a family history of sudden death or stroke)
- Mitral valve prolapse.

Answer 3   **Marks**

(a)   Hypoalbuminaemia <30 g/l
        Proteinuria > 3–5 g/24 hours
        Peripheral oedema   3

(b)   Fusion of the podocytes, with no other associated
        glomerular changes   2

(c)   24-hour urine collection – creatinine clearance and 24-hour
                                        protein
        Serum albumin
        USS of the kidneys, ureters and bladder
        Renal biopsy
        Therapeutic management –   high dose oral steroids
                                                   cyclophosphamide (in severe
                                                   cases)   5

Comment
Minimal change nephropathy is the commonest cause of an idiopathic nephrotic syndrome, accounting for 70–80% in children, 60% in adolescents and 25% in adults. It is not a true glomerulonephritis, and the characteristic fusion of the podocytes seen on electron microscopy is a non-specific sign which occurs in many other nephrotic states.
The pathogenesis of the disorder remains unclear, but it is thought to be an immune mediated disease as it responds so well to immunosuppression with high dose steroids or cyclophosphamide. It is associated with Hodgkin's lymphoma, and is seen to resolve with successful treatment of the lymphoma. In adolescents(>10 years old), and adults it is recommended the diagnosis is confirmed on renal biopsy. This is important as the disease does not progress to chronic renal failure and the patient may then be assured of a good prognosis.

Answer 4   **Marks**

(a)   Drugs – prescribed medications, e.g. gold salts and illicit
       drug abuse
       Infection, e.g. streptococcus, malaria
       Systemic vasculitides – SLE, PAN, Wegener's granulomatosis
       Diabetes mellitus
       Amyloidosis
       Allergic reactions   3

(b)   FBC, U+Es, glucose
       ESR
       Cholesterol
       Autoantibody screen – ANCA, ANF, rheumatoid factor
       24 hour urine collection for creatinine clearance and protein
       estimation
       USS of the kidneys
       Renal biopsy   5

(c)   Renal failure
       Renal vein thrombosis
       Sepsis   2

Comment
The glomerulonephritides are a heterogenous group of disorders, that are
characterized according to their pathological features under light and electron
microscopy, and by immunofluorescent staining. These features are a reflec-
tion of the glomerular damage that occurs due to deposition of immune
complexes or to antiglomerular basement membrane antibodies.
Common causes of the glomerulonephritides are:
•   Infection (Bacterial – streptococcus, leprosy, syphilis, infective
     endocarditis; Viral – EBV, HBV, HCV; Fungal – candidiasis;
     Parasitic – malaria, schistosomiasis)
•   Drugs (penicillamine, gold salts, ACE inhibitors)
•   Autoimmune (SLE, rheumatoid arthritis, thyroid disease)
•   Systemic vasculitides (Wegener's granulomatosis, PAN)
•   Malignancy (carcinoma of the lung, breast and colon, Hodgkin's
     disease)

Answer 5   **Marks**

(a)   Hyperkalaemia
       Renal failure
       Normochromic, normocytic anaemia   2

(b)   Poorly controlled diabetes mellitus
       Hypertension
       Recent addition of an ACE inhibitor   3

(c)   Hospital admission
       IV access
       IV 15–20 units of actrapid insulin with 40–50 ml of 50% dextrose
       Calcium resonium 15 g tds orally
       Consider IV calcium gluconate (cardioprotective)
       If the serum potassium does not fall, dialysis is required   5

Comment

Diabetic nephropathy principally arises due to microvascular disease, exacerbated by recurrent urinary tract infections and hypertension. The characteristic pathological change is nodular glomerulosclerosis, also called the Kimmelstiel–Wilson lesion. Progression of the nephropathy is readily divided into four categories:

- Hyperperfusion of the kidney associated with glomerular hypertrophy
- Microalbuminuria (this is a marker for both hypertension and the resultant damage to the renal parenchyma)
- Macroalbuminuria (>300 mg/24 hours – this occurs with progressive deterioration of the glomerular filtration and worsening hypertension)
- Frank renal failure (this may be associated with a nephrotic syndrome)

By maintaining tight normoglycaemic control with insulin, and adding an ACE inhibitor for hypertension and microalbuminuria, it has been shown that the progression of the disease may be retarded and, in some cases, even caused to regress.

Answer 6   **Marks**

(a)   Amyloidosis
       Drugs, e.g. NSAIDs and gold salts   2

(b)   USS of the kidneys
       Renal biopsy

Rectal biopsy for amyloid
24-hour urine collection for protein and creatinine clearance   3

(c)   Admit to a specialist renal unit
        Remove exacerbating factors, e.g. drugs
        Consider CAPD or haemofiltration depending on the degree
        of renal impairment
        Nutritional support – low protein diet
        Symptomatic relief of rheumatoid symptoms   5

Comment
Renal amyloidosis may arise through primary and secondary causes of amyloid.
It is mainly seen in AA amyloidosis but also occurs in 50% of AL amyloid.
AA amyloid commonly arises secondary to chronic inflammatory and
infective disorders, such as tuberculosis, rheumatoid arthritis, inflammatory
bowel disease, and malignancies, e.g. renal cell carcinoma.
Patients present with proteinuria, often to nephrotic levels, and postural
hypotension. Ultrasound scan will often reveal normal or enlarged kidneys,
even in end stage disease, due to the amyloid infiltration.
Diagnosis is made on renal or rectal biopsy, the latter being a more simple
procedure, with a high sensitivity. Histologically amyloid is characterized by
its ability to bind congo red, which gives it an apple green appearance under
polarized light.

Answer 7   **Marks**

(a)   Polyarteritis nodosa
        Henoch–Schönlein purpura
        Wegener's granulomatosis
        SLE   3

(b)   cANCA, pANCA, HBs antigen   2

(c)   Renal biopsy
        Renal angiography
        Skin biopsy
        Management –
                immunosuppression – azothioprine and cyclophosphamide
                antihypertensive therapy, e.g. ACE inhibitors, calcium
                channel blockers
                treatment of renal impairment – may require dialysis   5

Comment

The systemic vasculitides are a group of diseases characterized by inflammatory and degenerative changes within the blood vessel wall, causing a secondary systemic disorder, which commonly includes the kidney.

They are classified according to the size of the vessel they affect, and the presence or absence of associated granulomata.

Vessel size	Granuloma formation	No granuloma formation
Large	Giant cell arteritis	
	Takayasu's disease	
Medium		Polyarteritis nodosa
Small	Wegener's granulomatosis	Microscopic polyangiitis
	Churg Strauss syndrome	Henoch–Schönlein purpura

Polyarteritis nodosa, Wegener's granulomatosis, and microscopic polyangiitis classically cause vasculitic renal damage, with an associated glomerulonephritis and hypertension.

Polyarteritis is characterized by aneurysm formation within the renal vasculature, which is demonstrated by renal angiography. Unlike the other vasculitides in this group, polyarteritis has no specific immune marker, but in certain subgroups of patients there is an association with the HBs antigen.

Clinically, the disease normally presents with non-specific systemic features, such as myalgia, arthralgia, anorexia and low grade fever. However, in some cases its presentation is dramatic with myocardial infarction, CVA, or gastro-intestinal haemorrhage.

Treatment is similar for all of the systemic vasculitides, using high dose steroids and immunosuppressents, such as azothioprine and cyclophosphamide.

Answer 8   **Marks**

(a)   Normochromic, normocytic anaemia
       Hypoalbuminaemia
       Hypocalcaemia, hyperphosphataemia   3

(b)   Blood pressure (lying and standing)
       Urinalysis
       BM stix measurement   3

(c)   (i)   Anaemia – exclude Fe, B12 and
                folate deficiency
                blood transfusion – if symptomatic
                consider giving erythropoetin (EPO)

(ii)   Renal impairment – maintain good blood pressure
control
treat any underlying reversible or exacerbating
factors
will need dialysis, consider renal transplantation
(iii)   Hypocalcaemia – calcium supplements
(iv)   Hyperphosphateamia –
phosphate binders, e.g. aluminium hydroxide   4

Comment

Chronic renal failure is defined as an irreversible loss of renal function, characteristically associated with a substantial rise in urea and creatinine, a normochromic, normocytic anaemia, hypocalcaemia and hyperphosphataemia. The anaemia may be secondary to the underlying cause of the renal impairment, drug therapy or to the loss of renal erythropoetin production. The anaemic patient may require erythropoetin replacement, although only some patients benefit from this form of treatment, who are thought to be in a genetically determined subgroup.

The disturbances in calcium/phosphate metabolism result in several effects on the skeleton, known as renal osteodystrophy. Osteomalacia arises due to the defective renal hydroxylation of 25 hydroxy-cholecalciferol (25-OH,D3), which in turn leads to a reduced calcium absorption from the gut. Secondary hyperparathyroidism arises due to this chronic hypocalcaemia, which eventually causes tertiary hyperparathyroidism and leads to a rise in the calcium. Without treatment this hypercalcaemia leads to renal calcification, hypercalciuria, and further renal damage through stone formation.

Answer 9   **Marks**

(a)   Dehydration leading to pre-renal impairment
Thrombocytopaenia
Diabetes mellitus
Possible sepsis
Hyperosmolar pre-coma   3

(b)   Blood tests – clotting screen, including D-dimers and FDPs
Blood cultures
ABGs
MSU
ECG
CXR   4

(c)   Pre-renal: cardiogenic, hypovolaemic and septic shock
        Renal: tubulointerstitial nephritis, glomerulonephritis
        Post-renal (obstructive): stones, tumours, foreign bodies   3

Comment

Acute renal failure is characterized by a rapid deterioration in glomerular filtration rate, which clinically manifests itself as oligouria or anuria, and biochemically is reflected by worsening urea and creatinine.

It is usually classified into pre-renal, renal and (obstructive) post-renal causes:

*   Pre-renal – this results from hypoperfusion of the kidney due to renovascular disease or shock. If the cause remains uncorrected it causes acute tubular necrosis. Pre-renal failure is usually reversible providing the kidneys were functioning normally prior to the insult, and the causes are quickly diagnosed and treated.

*   Renal – examples include: acute tubular necrosis, glomerulonephritis, autoimmune disease (rheumatoid arthritis, SLE, systemic vasculitides), PAN, Wegener's granulomatosis, tubulointerstitial nephritis (sickle cell disease, NSAIDs, nephrotoxins), myoglobin, Bence–Jones proteins

*   Obstructive – this occurs due to internal obstruction or external compression of the urinary tract. External compression – prostatic enlargement, pelvic and rectal tumours, retroperitoneal fibrosis and lymphoma; Internal obstruction – ureteric stones, pelvicalyceal and ureteric tumours, bladder stones and tumours, foreign bodies

Answer 10   **Marks**

(a)   Anion gap $= [\,Na + K\,] - [\text{chloride} + \text{bicarbonate}]$
                  $= [\,134 + 3.1\,] - [\,114 + 12\,]$
                  $= 137.1 - 126$
                  $= 11.1$ (normal range 8–16 mmol/l)   3

(b)   Type I – sickle cell disease
      Type II – heavy metal toxicity
      Type IV – Addison's disease   3

(c)   Diabetic ketacidosis
      Lactic acidosis
      General management –   IV access
                            IV fluids
                            IV sliding scale of insulin

Treat underlying cause, e.g. sepsis
If new diagnosis –
    address associated risk factors
    diabetic education   4

Comment

Renal tubular acidosis is caused by a heterogenous group of disorders, and is characterized by hyperchloraemia, a normal anion gap and a metabolic (i.e. low bicarbonate) acidosis. There are three recognized variants, classified according to the abnormal tubule site.

Type I

Distal hypokalaemic hyperchloraemic acidosis – in this disorder the distal tubules are unable to secrete hydrogen (H^+) ions, which causes secondary hyperaldosteronism and results in the hypokalaemia and hyperchloraemia. Causes include:

- Autoimmune disease (SLE, CAH, Sjögren's syndrome)
- Drugs (NSAIDs, amphoterecin)
- Nephrocalcinosis (hyperparathyroidism)
- Obstructive nephropathy

Type II

Proximal hypokalaemic hyperchloraemic acidosis – the principal abnormality in this condition is the inability of the proximal tubules to reabsorb bicarbonate. It may be associated with a generalized defect of reabsorption, known as Fanconi syndrome, where amino acids, glucose and other ions are also lost in the urine.

Fanconi syndrome may be inherited as a rare autosomal recessive condition, but is more commonly acquired secondary to myeloma', heavy metal toxicity or drugs.

Type IV

Distal hyperkalaemic hyperchloraemic acidosis – this differs from type I in that there is a generalized distal tubular defect, with an associated reduction in the glomerular filtration rate, and the resulting hyperkalaemia may be life threatening.

Causes include mineralocorticoid deficiency in Addison's disease, adrenalectomy, diabetic nephropathy and obstructive nephropathy, and tubular resistance to mineralocorticoid effects, e.g. spironolactone. Type III is a rare condition which has elements of types I and II. It is now therefore not described as a separate entity.

CHAPTER 11: RHEUMATOLOGY AND CONNECTIVE TISSUE DISEASES ANSWERS

Answer 1   **Marks**

(a)   Rheumatoid arthritis   1

(b)   (i)   Sjögren's syndrome, scleromalacia
       (ii)   Rheumatoid nodules, vasculitic rash
       (iii)   Pleural effusion, rheumatoid nodules, pulmonary
               fibrosis
       (iv)   Pericarditis, pericardial effusions
       (v)   Chronic renal failure secondary to amyloid and drugs,
               e.g. gold salts   5
(c)   Patient education on the disease and complications
       Physiotherapy, occupational therapy and orthotist
       Drug therapy – paracetamol, NSAIDs
                      DMARDs (see comment)
                      cytotoxic agents, steroids
       Community support
       Surgical intervention   4

Comment

Rheumatoid arthritis is a common, chronic inflammatory arthropathy, which has multiple extra-articular manifestations. It has an autoimmune basis, with important genetic factors. It is associated with HLA DR1 and DR4, and has increased prevalence amongst certain racial groups, particularly some of the Native Indian tribes of North America. Environmental factors, including viral and bacterial infections, have also been implicated.

Immune markers for the disease include the classical rheumatoid factor, which is an IgM directed against IgG, and antinuclear factor(ANF). Both of these markers occur in several other rheumatological disorders and their exact role in pathogenesis remains unclear. High titres of the rheumatoid factor has prognostic implications and signifies increased likelihood of extra-articular manifestations.

Treatment of the disease initially is based on symptomatic relief with NSAIDs, but as the disease progresses the use of disease modifying agents of rheumatological disease (DMARDs) are used. This group of drugs, which includes D-penicillamine, gold salts, sulphasalazine and hydroxychloroquine, has been shown to retard the progression of the arthritic disease. However, they all tend to have multiple side effects, including renal impairment and bone marrow suppression, and their use should be supervised and reviewed regularly by a rheumatologist.

Chapter 11: Rheumatology and Connective Tissue Diseases Answers

Answer 2   **Marks**

(a)   Osteoarthritis of the right knee joint   1

(b)   Periarticular sclerosis
        Loss of the joint space
        Osteophyte formation
        Periarticular cysts
        Soft tissue swelling
        Healed fracture of the distal femur   5

(c)   Dietary advice, weight loss
        Analgesia
        Physiotherapy
        Walking aids as appropriate
        Consider surgical arthroplasty   4

Comment

Osteoarthritis is the commonest of all arthritides, its prevalence increasing with age, affecting 70–75% of the over 75s population. It is a disorder of the synovial joints, particularly affecting the weightbearing joints of the lower limbs. Pathologically it is characterized by loss of the articular cartilage and bony overgrowth. It has a multifactorial aetiology, the exact causes remaining unclear. Factors which predispose to development of the arthritis include:

- Familial tendency
- Hereditary disorders e.g. Ehlers–Danlos syndrome, the mucopolysaccharidoses
- Concomitant bone disease – Paget's bone disease, Perthe's disease, osteopetrosis, congenital dislocation of the hip (CDH)
- Repetitive occupational trauma e.g. professional football players, professional ballet dancers

Answer 3   **Marks**

(a)   Systemic lupus erythrematosus (SLE)   1

(b)   Anti-double stranded DNA (anti dsDNA) antibody
        Anti-smooth muscle (anti SM) antibody
        Anti-cardiolipin antibody
        Anti-Ro antibody
        Anti-La antibody
        Anti-U1 ribonuclear protein (anti-U1RNP) antibody   3

(c)   (i)   Butterfly (malar) rash, photosensitive rash, discoid lupus

        (ii)   Raynaud's phenomenon, vasculitic rash, venous thrombosis

        (iii)   Glomerulonephritis, chronic renal failure

        (iv)   Psychoses, seizures, peripheral neuropathy, cranial nerve palsies

        (v)   Coombs positive haemolytic anaemia, thrombocytopenia

        (vi)   Myopathy, non-erosive arthropathy   6

Comments

Systemic lupus erythrematosus (SLE) is the commonest of the collagen vascular disorders, with a prevalence of between 40–65:100,000. It is nine times more common in women and is particularly prevalent amongst Black women in the United States and the Caribbean. The peak incidence is between 20–40 years.

It is a multisystem disorder, but most commonly presents with musculoskeletal and cutaneous manifestations and symptoms. The skin changes may be part of the multisystem disorder or may be almost totally confined to the skin, known as discoid lupus. Several of the auto-antibodies which occur have been linked to specific syndromes within the disease. Anti-dsDNA has been linked to the development of nephritis, anti-Ro and anti-La to the photosensitivity syndrome, and the anti-cardiolipin antibody (the lupus anticoagulant), to the syndrome of recurrent miscarriage, thrombosis and thrombocytopaenia. The mainstay of treatment remains maintenance therapy with oral steroids, with the use of immunosuppressants, such as azothioprine and cyclophosphamide, being reserved for acute exacerbations of the disease.

Answer 4   **Marks**

(a)   Raynaud's phenomenon   1

(b)   Calcinosis
        Raynaud's phenomenon
        Oesophageal dysmotility
        Sclerodactyly
        Telangiectasia
        The syndrome is now termed limited cutaneous systemic sclerosis   4

(c)   Educate the patient and family about the disease and prognosis
        Raynaud's – treatment and prophylaxis
        Skin care

Immunosuppression
Nutritional support – may require gastrostomy feeding if
dysphagia is severe
Treatment of specific complications –
    pulmonary fibrosis, pulmonary hypertension
    chronic renal impairment   5

Comment
Progressive systemic sclerosis, (previously called scleroderma), is a multisystem connective tissue disease which principally presents with skin changes
and Raynaud's phenomenon. It is 3–4 times more common in women and its
peak incidence is between 30–60 years. It is now subdivided into limited and
diffuse cutaneous disease.
The limited disease, previously termed the CREST syndrome, is the more
common. The associated Raynaud's phenomenon, whereby the digits become
painful and progress through several colour stages, i.e. white to cyanosed to
red, on exposure to the cold, requires both prophylaxis and treatment.
Avoidance of cold exposure and protection against the cold with heated
gloves and socks is the main prophylaxis. Calcium channel blockers, ACEIs
and 5-HT2 inhibitors are used in long term therapy, with a prostacyclin
infusion reserved for the more acute cases.
The diffuse disease affects the lungs, heart, bowels and kidneys most
commonly. Pulmonary fibrosis causes increasing respiratory failure, leading
to pulmonary hypertension. Unlike the limited disease, the entire bowel may
be affected by dysmotility problems, and as the disease progresses this will
require increasing nutritional support. Cardiac manifestations include
cardiomyopathy, myocarditis and pericardial effusions. Several immunosuppressants are used in the treatment of the disease, but as yet, none have
been shown to influence the prognosis.

Answer 5   **Marks**

(a)   Gout   1

(b)   Serum uric acid
        X-ray of the left foot
        Examine joint aspirate under polarized light microscopy for
        negatively bifringent crystals   3

(c)   Risk factors –
        increased purine turnover – leukaemia, psoriasis

increased purine synthesis – Lesch–Nyhan syndrome
alcohol excess
drugs – thiazide and loop diuretics, low dose aspirin
toxins – lead
Drug therapy –
    NSAIDs, e.g. indomethacin – renal impairment
    colchicine – diarrhoea
    allopurinol – worsens acute gouty episode   6

Comment

Gout is the commonest of the crystal deposition disorders, and is caused by abnormal uric acid metabolism, leading to the deposition of sodium urate in the joints, soft tissues and renal tract. It presents in middle age and is more common in men, and the upper social classes. In most patients the disease is idiopathic, although there are several predisposing conditions.

Hyperuricaemia is a marker for the disease, but is 10 times more common than symptomatic gout. The disease leads to an erosive arthropathy, commonly effecting the distal interphalangeal joints of the fingers and the interphalangeal joints of the toes. It should always be considered in the differential diagnosis of an acute monoarthritis.

The treatment of gout is divided for the acute and chronic disease. In an acute attack, NSAIDs or colchicine are used. Long term therapy is aimed at reducing the risk factors, treating any predisposing conditions and the use of allopurinol. Allopurinol should not be given within 4–6 weeks of an acute episode as it may precipitate another acute episode.

Answer 6   Marks

(a)   Polymyalgia rheumatica
       Giant cell arteritis   2

(b)   Rheumatoid arthritis
       Multiple myeloma   2

(c)   (i)   Temporal artery biopsy   2
       (ii)   High dose steroids (50–60 mg o.d.)   1
       (iii) Angina, temporal headaches, stroke
              Sudden blindness
              Jaw claudication   3

Comment

Polymyalgia rheumatica is an idiopathic disorder which presents between the ages of 50–70. It classically produces an ESR of >100, and clinically is associated with early morning stiffness of the shoulder and pelvic girdle muscle, which improves slowly with exertion. There is no definitive investigation for this disorder and anyone with suspected disease should be started on a trial of oral steroids. These may be slowly reduced according to the clinical response and the reduction in the ESR. Most patients are able to stop the steroids within 2–3 years of the diagnosis being made, but relapses are quite common.

Temporal arteritis may be regarded as the opposite end of a spectrum with polymyalgia. It is caused by a giant cell arteritis, which can affect facial, cerebral, cardiac and mesenteric arteries, and thus produces a varied group of presenting features, including jaw claudication with talking or eating, angina, and sudden blindness due to involvement of the retinal artery. It is therefore essential to start steroid therapy in any suspected cases, and attempts should be made to obtain histological confirmation by temporal artery biopsy. There is a 48-hour window between starting the steroids and obtaining the biopsy, before the steroids affect the histological changes and make the biopsy valueless.

Answer 7   **Marks**

(a)   Wegener's granulomatosis
      Classical triad: upper and lower respiratory tract, and renal
      involvement   2

(b)   Rheumatoid arthritis
      Polyarteritis nodosa
      Streptococcal infection
      Drug allergy
      Mixed essential cryoglobulinaemia   4

(c)   FBC, clotting screen, ESR
      cANCA, and other autoantibodies
      CXR
      Bronchoscopy and biopsy
      Renal ultrasound scan
      Renal biopsy
      Cyclophosphamide is the drug of choice   4

Comment
Wegener's granulomatosis is a small vessel vasculitis associated with the formation of granulomata. It remains an idiopathic disease, but the relatively recent identification of the autoantibody cANCA, and more precisely the anti-proteinase 3 antibodies, have led to an improvement in both understanding of the pathogenesis and the treatment of the disorder. These antibodies are present in 80–85% of cases and are immune markers for the disease. They are also used to follow the success of therapy and to monitor disease activity.

Clinically the disorder is characterized by the classical triad above, but also produces multiple systemic features, including malaise, fever, myalgia, and polyarthritis. Skin and eye involvement are common, and the disease may also affect the central and peripheral nervous systems, causing hypothalamic-pituitary dysfunction and mononeuritis multiplex.

Treatment of the disease initially includes cyclophosphamide and steroids, these may be reduced slowly, depending on the response. Other cytotoxics such as azothioprine may be used instead of cyclophosphamide.

Answer 8	**Marks**

(a) Osteoporosis — 1

(b) (i) Poor dietary calcium intake during adolescence
Premature menopause (as in this case)
Lack of weightbearing exercise
Prolonged amenorrhoea – long distance runners, anorexia
nervosa — 3

  (ii) Medications – Analgesia
Cyclical bisphosphonates
Hormone replacement therapy
Calcitonin — 3

(c) Advice to her daughter should include –
regular weightbearing exercise
maintain a good diet with adequate calcium intake
avoid alcohol excess and smoking — 3

Comment
Osteoporosis is a common metabolic bone disorder that principally occurs in post-menopausal women. Pathologically it is characterized by a decrease in bone mass without a change in the bone's cellular composition.

Peak bone mass occurs in the early 20s, and its subsequent rate of loss is dependent on genetic and environmental factors, as well as intercurrent illnesses. It is therefore important that during the growth period of childhood and adolescence, individuals maintain adequate nutrition and particularly 'load' their diet with calcium. All other risk factors should also be addressed. Post-menopausal women should be offered hormone replacement therapy (HRT), although at present it is unclear as to how long this should continue. Women suffering a premature menopause, either due to autoimmune disease, or surgical removal of the ovaries, are particularly at risk, not only of developing osteoporosis but also ischaemic heart disease, and they too should be placed on HRT.

The diagnosis is confirmed by X-ray findings and DEXA scan, which may also be used in assessing a patient's risk of developing the disease.

Confirmed cases should receive cyclical sodium etidronate, a bisphosphonate, which inhibits osteoclastic bone resorption, and is particularly useful in vertebral bone disease. Acute cases require analgesia and may benefit from the use of calcitonin, which has been shown to improve outcome and has some analgesic effect.

Answer 9   **Marks**

(a)   Increased bone turnover with associated remodelling and
defective mineralization   2

(b)   X-rays of the right hip, pelvis and lumbar spine
Serum calcium, phosphate and alkaline phosphatase
Urinary hydroxyproline   3

(c)   Complications – bone pain
                        vertebral collapse and resultant paraplegia
                        'high output' cardiac failure
                        deafness
                        osteosarcoma
Therapeutic management – adequate analgesia
                                      bedrest
                                      bisphosphonates, calcitonin or
                                      mithramycin   5

Comment
Paget's disease of the bone is a common metabolic bone disorder, which occurs after the age of 40. Its prevalence increases with age, particularly in women. The disease is idiopathic, but latest theories propose a viral agent, due

to the discovery of viral like inclusions seen within the osteoclasts. Several viruses have been studied including RSV, measles, and canine distemper virus. Clinically it presents with pain and bony deformity, classically causing anterior bowing of the tibia and enlargement of the skull. The bones may feel warm due to increased vascularity, and pathological fractures may occur, particularly in the pelvis and the vertebrae, where subsequent collapse can lead to spinal cord compression. The progression to osteosarcoma is rare occurring in only 1% of cases. Investigations will reveal a normal calcium and phosphate with an elevated alkaline phosphatase, which reflects the increased osteoblastic activity. A raised calcium, should alert the physician to the possibility of concurrent malignancy, hyperparathyroidism or prolonged immobility. Patients should be treated with bisphosphonates, which decrease the excessive bone turnover. Calcitonin is used for bony pain and in the post-operative period of patients undergoing joint arthroplasty, where it reduces bleeding. Rarely, mithramicin is also used.

Answer 10   **Marks**

(a)   HLA B27
       Reiter's syndrome, psoriasis, inflammatory bowel disease   3

(b)   Ankylosis of the vertebrae with syndesmophyte formation –
       'bamboo spine'
       Calcification of the spinous ligaments
       Sacro-ileitis   3

(c)   (i)   Anterior uveitis
       (ii)   Conduction system fibrosis
       (iii)   Upper zone pulmonary fibrosis
       (iv)   Atlanto-axial subluxation with resulting cord
                compression and tetraplegia   4

Comment

Ankylosing spondylitis is a progressive inflammatory disorder, which is particularly prevalent in young men. It causes severe back pain which is classically worse in the morning and improves with exercise. Progression of the disease leads to a gross reduction in the range of movement of the cervical and lumbar spine, causing the patient to develop a marked kyphosis. This, in association with the loss of the lumbar lordosis, produces the classical 'question mark' posture. Extra-articular manifestations are common and are as follows:

- Pulmonary (apical fibrosis; although commonly quoted this is in fact relatively rare)
- Cardiac (conduction system fibrosis, leading to varying degrees of heart block. An ascending aortitis occurs with associated aortic valve regurgitation pericarditis and cardiomyopathy may also occur)
- Eyes (anterior uveitis, this occurs in 25–30% of cases)
- Renal (secondary amyloidosis may occur causing chronic renal failure)

Treatment should include NSAIDs for analgesia and more importantly a physiotherapy programme, which retards the spinal deformity. In patients where NSAIDs are ineffective, sulphasalazine is used, but the use of other immunosuppressants have failed to influence the long term prognosis.

Answer 11   **Marks**

(a)   Reiter's syndrome
       Urethritis, conjunctivitis and arthritis   2

(b)   Chlamydia Spp
       Campylobacter jejuni
       Shigella
       Yersinia   3

(c)   Investigations –
               FBC, blood cultures
               HLA typing
               Urethral swabs for chlamydia and other STDs
               Syphilis serology
               Aspiration of knee joint for microbiological review
               Consider HIV test with pre-test counselling
       Therapeutic management –
               appropriate antibiotics, e.g. ciprofloxacin
               bedrest; non-weightbearing on affected leg
               counselling and education about the disease
               contact tracing of any sexual contacts   5

Comment

Reiter's syndrome is a characterized by the triad of conjunctivitis, urethritis and a reactive arthritis. The associated arthritis is aseptic and usually affects a single joint, particularly of the lower limb. The disease is strongly associated with HLA B27, and is usually precipitated by a gastrointestinal or urogenital infection. The syndrome has several other acute manifestations, including anterior uveitis, circinate balanitis, achilles tendonitis, plantar fascitis, and keratoderma blenorrhagicum. Clinically the disease may have one of three courses. An acute illness with complete resolution, a prolonged single episode, which lasts over six months and requires immunosuppressants, and a recurring, episodic disorder, which may be due to reactivation with a new infection or solely due to the original illness. It is important that the patient is made aware of the possibility of recurrence.

CHAPTER 12: PSYCHIATRY ANSWERS

Answer 1   **Marks**

(a)   **C** – have you ever felt you should **C**ut down on your
             drinking?
       A – have people **A**nnoyed you by criticizing your drinking?
       G – have you ever felt bad or **G**uilty about your drinking?
       E – have you ever had to take a drink first thing in the
             morning to steady your nerve or get rid of a hangover?
             (**E**ye opener)   4

(b)   MCV
       LFTs and gamma glutamyl transferase   2

(c)   Obtain a full history from the patient and wife – separately if
       required
       Screening tests
       Patient must accept there is a problem before further help can
       be given
       Acute withdrawl – diazepam and psychological support
       Long term support –
             alcohol abuse self help groups, e.g. Alcoholics Anonymous,
             deterrent drugs
             psychiatric help may be required   4

Comment

Alcohol abusers or problem drinkers are an extremely heterogenous group of
individuals, crossing all social and economic barriers. It is estimated that
approximately 1:20 adults in the UK are problem drinkers, with 25% of
inpatients estimated to have alcohol-related problems. Depite the recent
changes recommended by the Department of Health, the medical community
still regards the 'safe' limits for alcohol consumption to be 14 units/week for
a woman and 21 units/week for a man (where one unit is equal to a single
measure of spirits, a glass of wine, or a half pint of beer).

Problem drinking causes psychological, physical and social problems, which
are dose-related. Physical and psychological dependence will cause withdrawal symptoms within 12–24 hours of abstinence. The physical symptoms
include palpitations, tremor, sweating, retching, vomiting and seizures.

Several syndromes arise due to the direct effects of the alcohol or its withdrawal:

*   Delirium tremens – this presents on alcohol withdrawl with altered
     level of consciousness, confusion, agitation and tremor. In extreme

forms there may be associated aural and visual hallucination and paranoid delusions
- Korsakov's syndrome – characterized by short term memory loss and confabulation
- Wernicke's encephalopathy – this is associated with confusion, nystagmus and VIth nerve palsy

The most difficult part of treatment of the problem drinker is the acceptance that there is a problem, and abstinence. Once this has been achieved, physical withdrawl may be attempted, usually aided by the use of diazepam (chlormethiazole is still used in most hospitals, but it remains an expensive and relatively poor drug for this situation). Nutritional deficiencies, particularly vitamin B complex, should be corrected, parenterally if necessary.

Answer 2   **Marks**

(a)   Elderly, male
      Long suicide note
      Recent bereavement   3

(b)   Method of attempt
      Precautions against being discovered
      Seeking help prior to or after the attempt
      Planning of the attempt   3

(c)   Management – Initial therapy –
                Protection of the airway, IV access
                Blood tests – FBC, U+Es, glucose, LFTs, clotting
                            paracetamol and salicylate levels
                            (serum should be saved for other drug
                            levels, e.g. tricyclic antidepressants)
                Stomach washout (with anaesthetist management of
                the airway)
                Specific treatment directed against the tablets he has taken
      Psychiatric therapy –
                must be admitted as this was a serious suicide attempt
                antidepressants
                bereavement counselling   4

Comment

Non-fatal deliberate self-harm or parasuicide has dramatically increased in incidence over the last century, now leading to almost 100,000 acute admissions per year in the UK. The commonest method, accounting for 90% of cases, is self-poisoning, principally with paracetamol, aspirin, minor tranquillizers and antidepressents.

Self-poisoning is more prevalent amongst young women particularly in lower social classes, although recent trends have shown increased rates amongst young men.

Important factors to consider in the history of a patient presenting with non-fatal deliberate self-harm are:

* Family or personal history of previous suicide atempts
* Family or personal history of psychiatric illnesss
* Personal relationship problems
* Employment stress or unemployment
* Recent bereavement
* Social isolation
* Financial problems
* Concurrent serious or chronic illness

It is estimated that 20–25% of self-poisoners will make further attempts. This is increased if there is evidence of alcohol or drug abuse, psychiatric illness, social isolation and unemployment.

Answer 3   **Marks**

(a)   Anorexia nervosa
        Body weight reduced by 10–15% of expected or previous
        weight
        Self induced weight loss by avoidance of fattening foods   3

(b)   Body mass index   (BMI) = $\dfrac{\text{weight in kilos}}{(\text{height in metres})^2}$

        BMI   = 30 / 1.60
               = 30 / 2.56
               = 11.72 (normal range = 20–26)   3

(c)   Investigations –   FBC and MCV
                                      U+Es
                                      albumin
                                      calcium, phosphate and magnesium
                                      B12, folate and ferretin
                                      TFTs
                                      FSH / LH
                                      antiendomesial antibody

Management –   confirm the diagnosis by history and
                         investigation
                         address underlying psychological or
                         social problems
                         in mild cases – regular follow up and
                         dietary advice
                         more severe cases – admit to specialist unit;
                         nutritional support, psychiatric therapy   4

Comment

The major eating disorders are a product of modern Western society and have become prevalent only in the last 20–30 years. They are made up of the two extremes in body form, anorexia and bulimia nervosa at one end of the spectrum and obesity with associated psychological problems at the other.

Anorexia nervosa is a complex disorder that usually occurs in adolescence and early adulthood, and is particularly prevalent in girls of this age. Bulimia is recognised as a variant of anorexia, with self-induced vomiting associated with intractable over eating. Both are considered to be primarily psychiatric disorders, with psychological, emotional and environmental causative factors. The diagnostic criteria for anorexia nervosa were defined by the ICD-10:-

(1) Body weight maintained at 15% or more below that expected, or in pre-pubertal patients, failure to make expected weight gain during the growth period.

(2) The weight loss is self-induced by avoidance of fattening foods and is associated with at least one of the following – self-induced vomiting or purging, excessive exercise, the use of appetite suppressants or diuretics.

(3) The dread of fatness is viewed as an intrusive, overvalued idea, and there is self-imposition of a low weight threshold. This is accompanied by amenorrhoea in the female and loss of libido and impotence in the male. There is also delayed or arrested puberty in pre-pubertal patients.

Answer 4   Marks

(a) (i) Opiate overdose
           Immediate management –   intravenous access
                                     protection of the airway
                                     IV naloxone   3
    (ii) Pin point pupils will confirm the diagnosis   1

(b)   Intravenous – known as 'mainlining'
       Smoking/inhalation – known as 'chasing the dragon'   2

(c)   (i)   Neurological – agitation, parasthesia and dilated pupils

       (ii)   Psychological – depression, craving

       (iii)   Gastrointestinal – diarrhoea, vomiting, abdominal cramps

       (iv)   Dermatological – sweating, 'goose bumps'   4

Comment

Opiates remain one of the most commonly abused group of drugs, mainly in the form of heroin. It may be injected, smoked or even taken in tablet form. Psychological and physical dependence are common in regular use, but unlike many drugs tolerance means that addicts must increase their intake to maintain the same level of effect.

Withdrawal, commonly known as 'cold turkey', because of the associated shivering and goose bumps, is extremely unpleasant, but is rarely life threatening. Both physical and psychological symptoms are prominent. Medically supervised withdrawal, involves replacement of the heroin with methadone, (which itself may become the focus of addiction), and slow reduction in the dose. This period should involve a specialist unit, to provide community, social and psychological support.

It must be remembered that various drugs have been abused throughout history, and what is regarded as illicit to one culture, remains acceptable to another. Although opiates, hallucinogenics, stimulants and sedatives remain illegal in the Western world, many more people suffer illness and death each year through alcohol and nicotine related disease. Health care professionals must remain impartial and resist being judgemental.

Answer 5   **Marks**

(a)   Reactive depression – bereavement reaction

        Loss of interest in person and environment

        Loss of appetite, weight loss

        Insomnia, early morning waking   3

(b)   Psychotherapy – including bereavement counselling

        Cognitive therapy

        In severe cases – electroconvulsive therapy (ECT)   2

(c)   Tricyclic antidepressants, e.g. amitriptyline – anticholinergic side effects, e.g. dry mouth

        MAOIs, e.g. phenelzine – causes a hypertensive crisis with amines

5HT uptake inhibitors – fluoxetine, paroxetine –
hyponatraemia   5

Comment
Depression may be divided into primary or endogenous and secondary or
reactive. Clinically patients may present with features of both, and this often
makes the division academic. The table below shows the features of each.

	Primary	**Secondary**
Identifiable precipitating factor	no	yes
Premorbid personality	stable	often predisposing personality trait
Environmental influences	unresponsive to environmental influences	fluctuates according to environmental factors

The somatic features are common to both, e.g. anorexia, diurnal mood, early
morning waking, insomnia.
Therapy is divided into pharmacological and psychological treatment. In mild
to moderate depression patients often do as well with psychoanalysis and
counselling as with drug therapy. In more serious cases, however, the patients
often require both forms of therapy and in very severe cases, may also require
ECT.

Answer 6   **Marks**

(a)   Auditory hallucination
        Delusional perception   2

(b)   Premorbid – unemployment, poor home environment
        Presenting – insidious onset, multiple first rank symptoms   4

(c)   Medical therapy –   acute – antipsychotics, e.g.
                             chlorpromazine
                             chronic – depot injection of a
                             phenothiazine (usually fortnightly)
        Psychiatric therapy – psychiatrists and community
        psychiatric nurses
        Multidisciplinary team – psychologists, counsellors and family
        education and support   4

Comment

Schizophrenia is a common psychotic illness, with a prevalence of 2–4 per 1000 of the population. Both environmental and genetic factors have been implicated in its aetiology, but the exact mechanisms remain unclear. Several abnormalities of neurotransmitters within the central nervous system have been identified, including excess dopaminergic activity and abnormal mono-amine oxidase levels.

Schneider, in the early part of the 20th century, coined the phrase 'first rank symptoms'. Exhibition of these symptoms at presentation, in the absence of other organic causes, particularly drugs, is highly specific to the diagnosis. These are:

* Auditory hallucination
* Thought withdrawal, insertion or interruption
* Thought broadcasting
* Delusional perception
* Somatic passivity
* External control of emotions

Prognosis is variable, and depends on several factors. A relatively good prognosis can be expected, when the illness develops acutely, has a clear precipitating factor, and the patient's premorbid personality and environment were stable.

Answer 7   **Marks**

(a)   Mania
      Manic depressive or bipolar affective disorder   3

(b)   Increased energy and activity
      Lack of sleep
      Grandiose ideas and delusions of grandeur
      Increased libido   3

(c)   Haloperidol – parkinsonism, confusion, sedation, neuroleptic
      malignant syndrome
      Lithium – nephrogenic diabetes insipidus, confusion, coma,
      tremor, vomiting and diarrhoea   4

Comment

Mania is an abnormal state characterized by an elevation of mood, increased energy and activity and ideas of self-importance. It presents with a spectrum of symptoms, ranging from a mild to moderate disorder, termed hypomania, to a florid psychotic state. Patients may fluctuate between symptoms of mania and episodes of depression, known as a bipolar affective disorder. This is more common than isolated mania, and is more prevalent in women than men. More unusually, patients may exhibit symptoms of both depression and mania at the same time, termed mixed affective disorder. Clinically, patients have rapid or forced speech, with 'flight of ideas'. They also express grandiose ideas, and occasionally have delusions of grandeur. Acutely, patients require admission to a psychiatric unit, and antipsychotics. Lithium is also used in the treatment of acute mania and in long term maintenance therapy. It has a narrow therapeutic window and levels must be carefully monitored. Toxicity initially causes blurred vision, diarrhoea, nausea and vomiting, progressing to confusion, seizures and coma. Other side effects include hypothyroidism, hypokalaemia and rarely, chronic renal impairment.

Answer 8   **Marks**

(a)   Dys-social, psychopathic or sociopathic   2

(b)   Personality disorder is an exaggeration of personality traits
        which lead to suffering by the individual or others
        Examples – paranoid, schizoid, emotionally unstable   5

(c)   Genetic factors
        Developmental factors –   environmental factors
                                    constitutional disorders
        Psychological factors   3

Comment
Personality disorder is a complex concept in which there is an exaggeration of the normal personality traits. The ICD-10 classified the disorder into the following subtypes:
*   Anxious or avoidant
*   Dependent
*   Dys-social or psychopathic
*   Emotionally unstable
*   Histrionic
*   Obsessive compulsive or anankastic
*   Paranoid
*   Schizoid
The importance of various factors that influence the development of these abnormal personalities remains unclear. It is known from work with mono-

zygotic twins that genetic factors do play a role, as do constitutional factors. Normal personality is formed principally through psychodynamic and psychological influences during childhood. Thus, in predisposed individuals, it is believed that abnormal influences cause the development of these abnormal personality disorders.

Therapy is based on individual and group psychotherapy, with behavioural modification and social skills training. However in dys-social disorders, individuals are often violent and they require treatment in specialist, secure units with various psychotherapeutic and behavioural approaches employed.

Answer 9	**Marks**

(a)   Obsessive-compulsive disorder   2

(b)   Neurosis – is an inappropriate emotional or behavioural
response to a perceived stressor
Examples – anxiety states, phobic conditions   4

(c)   Treatment principally involves behavioural psychotherapy,
i.e. response prevention; modelling and confrontation
Medications, e.g. tricyclic antidepressants   4

Comment

Unlike the psychotic patient, the neurotic never loses contact with reality, and has normal mental functioning. Obsessive-compulsive disorders arise due to obsessional, unwanted thoughts, which the patient cannot resist even though they realize they are wrong. The repetitive rituals or actions they perform as a result of these thoughts are known as compulsions. If these compulsions are resisted the patient often becomes depressed or anxious.

Therapy for these patients is principally based on behavioural psychotherapy. Response prevention is where the patient is encouraged to initiate self-restraint when faced with compulsive actions, e.g. in the case above, the man would be asked to delay washing his hands, and would have someone observe and encourage him whilst he did so. Initially the observer is the therapist or nurse, but with time a family member may take over this role.

Modelling is the process whereby the therapist demonstrates (models) to the patient that their compulsive thoughts are not based on rational ideas. This may be combined with confrontation, where the patient is repeatedly exposed to a situation which would normally initiate their compulsive behaviour. The idea being that with time the anxiety is greatly reduced, so the stimulus is lessened. Some patients benefit from antidepressants, which gives some credence to the theory that these disorders arise due to abnormal 5HT and dopamine activity. The prognosis is usually good, but is worsened with insidious onset or chronic presentations.

CHAPTER 13: CARE OF THE ELDERLY ANSWERS

Answer 1   **Marks**

(a)   Dementia – probably multi-infarct disease   1

(b)   Name   Name of the prime minister
       Address for recall   Name of the monarch
       Date of birth   Date of the WW1 or WW2
       Place   Recognition of two people
       Year   Count backwards from 20 to 1   5

(c)   Social history –   housing
                             mobility +/– aids
                             continence/toilet facilities
                             ADLs
                             present carers and how they are coping
                             present social services input
       Multidisciplinary team – physiotherapist, occupational therapist
                                 dietitian
                                 continence advisor
                                 district nurse liaison
                                 dementia support team
                                 social worker
Consider day care, luncheon clubs and respite admissions to help
carers   4

Comment
Dementia is defined as 'a syndrome of the loss of intellectual function and
memory, which leads to the breakdown of normal daily functioning, whilst
the level of consciousness remains unaffected'.
The prevalence increases exponentially after the age of 65, affecting 3–4% of
those aged 65, increasing to 20–25% at 80.
75% of cases are caused by primary degenerative dementia, which includes
senile dementia of the Alzheimer's type (SDAT), and multi-infarct dementia
(MID). Although these are two separate clinical and pathological entities,
many patients have a combination of the two.
Classical Alzheimer's disease occurs in the under 65s, and is characterized
pathologically by the presence of neurofibrillary tangles in the cerebral
cortex. It has a relatively malignant course, with rapid deterioration of mental
abilities and premature death; in SDAT, which occurs in the over 65s, there is
a more benign course.
Multi-infarct disease, classically gives a stepwise progressive loss in

intellectual function, the steps reflecting multiple cerebrovascular events that vary in their size and clinical effect. The patients often have multiple risk factors for atherosclerotic disease.

Although the other causes of dementia account for only 15–25% of cases, they are important to exclude, as they can on occasion be reversible:

- Infective – AIDs dementia complex (progressive multifocal leuco-encephalopathy, cerebral toxoplasmosis and cryptococcus infection), tertiary syphilis, Creutzfeld–Jakob disease
- Primary neurological disease – Lewy body dementia, Pick's disease, multiple sclerosis, Parkinson's disease, progressive supranuclear palsy
- Metabolic – chronic dialysis, chronic hypoglycaemic episodes, B12 deficiency
- Malignancy – primary and secondary tumours
- Endocrine disease – hypothyroidism, Addison's disease, acromegaly
- Drugs – chronic use of barbiturates, lithium, cimetidine, anti-cholinergics
- Toxins – alcohol, heavy metals, e.g. lead, mercury

Answer 2   **Marks**

(a)   Right basal pneumonia
        Diabetic pre-coma
        Atrial fibrillation – may be secondary to myocardial
        infarction
        Possible collapse secondary to MI, CVA, or arrhythmia,
        with associated aspiration pneumonia   1

(b)   Haematological –   FBC, U+Es, glucose, CK-MB, blood
                             cultures
        Non-haemotological – ECG, CXR, MSU, ABGs
                             consider CT head scan   5

(c)   Management –   IV access
                             Broad spectrum antibiotics
                             IV insulin sliding scale
                             Treatment of fast AF – digoxin or amiodarone
                             NGT – consider enteral feeding
                             Subcutaneous heparin   4

Comment

The acute confusional state or delirium, is a common presentation in the elderly. As in this case, the elderly patient often presents with multiple pathologies, and it may be difficult to decide the primary disorder and the secondary sequelae. It is therefore important to consider all of the possible diagnoses and 'cover' the patient for the most serious or life threatening. In the care of the elderly patient, it should be remembered that it is the patient's premorbid health that is the main determinant of outcome and not their chronological age. In all cases a sense of perspective must be maintained, and one must always try to be appropriate in one's treatment.

Causes of acute confusional states include:

- Sepsis – commonly due to chest and urinary tract infections. However, many patients present with non-specific symptoms and deteriorate rapidly. Therefore antibiotics are often given empirically in the sick elderly patient, not only to cover primary sepsis but also the near inevitable secondary sepsis that occurs in this group of patients.
- Neurological – TIAs, CVAs, subdural haematoma, epilepsy, intracerebral tumours – benign and malignant
- Metabolic – hyper and hypoglycaemia, hyponatraemia, hypercalcaemia, uraemia
- Drugs – sedatives, diuretics, neuroleptics, antiepiletics, digoxin
- Endocrine – Addison's disease, hypothyroidism
- Others – paraneoplastic syndrome, GI bleeds, hypoxia, hypercapnia

Answer 3   Marks

(a)   Simple falls, e.g. poor mobility
Postural hypotension secondary to medications
Anaemia secondary to aspirin
Arrhythmias – IHD, medications, electrolyte derangement
Brainstem TIAs   3

(b)   FBC, U+Es, digoxin level
Lying/standing blood pressure
24-hour ambulatory ECG monitoring
Consider OGD and EEG   3

(c)   ACEI – first dose hypotension, dry cough, worsening
renal impairment
Loop diuretics – postural hypotension, hyponatraemia,
hypokalaemia

Digoxin – arrhythmia, nausea and vomiting
Aspirin – peptic ulceration   4

Comment

Falls are a common cause of morbidity and are markers of mortality in the elderly, with 50% of those sustaining a fractured neck of femur, dying within one year. Common causes include:

*   'Simple' falls (these have no identifiable causes, and may be due to a combination of environmental and constitutional factors)
*   Environmental (loose carpets, unstable furniture, uneven/slippery floors)
*   Cardiovascular (tachy/bradyarrhythmia; complete heart block, significant aortic stenosis, silent myocardial ischaemia)
*   Neurological (TIAs, CVAs, epilepsy, Parkinson's disease, vertebro-basilar insufficiency, carotid hypersensitivity)
*   Drugs (antihypertensives, antidysrrhythmics, oral hypoglycaemics, psychotropics)
*   Toxins (alcohol)
*   Other causes of postural hypotension (low output heart failure, autonomic dysfunction)

Constitutional factors which increase the likelihood of falling include visual and auditory impairment, dementia, muscular weakness, nutritional deficiency, chronic systemic disease, and age related changes in postural and gait reflexes.

Answer 4   **Marks**

(a)   Untreated urinary tract infection
        Worsening dementia
        Poor mobility
        Medications, e.g. diuretics   3

(b)   U+Es, glucose
        MSU
        Urine cytology
        USS of bladder, ureters and kidneys
        Flexible cystoscopy   3

(c)   Simple measures –   incontinence pads
                            ensure regular toileting and easy access to
                            toilet facilities

	review medications – dose and frequency	
	treat underlying infections; atrophic vaginitis	
Others –	anticholinergics, e.g. oxybutinin	
	surgical correction of urological or	
	gynaecological abnormalities	
	long term catheterization	4

Comment

Urinary incontinence is a common reason for admission in the elderly, and is deemed to be one of the four 'geriatric giants', with immobility, confusion and falls. Chronic or recurring incontinence may be divided into four categories:

• **Stress** – this is characterized by the loss of small volumes of urine, with increases in the intra-abdominal pressure, e.g. with laughing or coughing. It is principally caused by bladder outflow tract and pelvic floor weakness, and usually requires surgical correction.

• **Urge** – this is caused by detrusor muscle instability, which may be associated with local urogenital disease – cystitis, urethritis or tumours; neurological conditions – dementia, CVA, spinal cord compression.

• **Overflow** – this is usually associated with mechanical pressures on the bladder outflow tract causing urinary retention, with associated secondary overflow, e.g. obstruction – prostatic enlargement, urethral stricture, tumours; neuropathic bladder – diabetes, multiple sclerosis, spinal cord compression.

• **Functional** – this is due to an inability to reach the toilet through physical or cognitive impairment, e.g. confusional states, arthritis, depression, medications.

Reversible causes should be addressed, but if incontinence continues then conservative measures should be considered, as listed above.

Answer 5   **Marks**

(a)   Premorbid health – malnutrition, pre-existing systemic disease
         Pathological fall – MI, arrhythmia, CVA
         Operative complications, significant blood loss, prolonged
         anaesthesia
         Post-operative complications – sepsis, confusion, anaemia,
         depression   3

(b)   FBC, U+Es, glucose, TFTs, calcium
         pre- and post-operative ECGS
         CXR

lying and standing blood pressure
consider – 24-hour tape, CT head scan   3

(c)   Check all the above investigations treating any reversible
        factors, e.g. UTI
        ensure adequate analgesia whilst trying to avoid polypharmacy
        multidisciplinary input – physiotherapy, occupational therapy
                                    – social workers
        continue to monitor progress, and liaise with orthopaedic
        surgeons   4

Comment
The speed by which patients recover from surgery depends on preoperative,
operative and post-operative complications. Elderly patients with increased
co-morbidity and polypharmacy often take a little longer than younger
patients and therefore may require more intense preoperative planning to
maximize their health and post-operative assistance.

Fit, elderly patients do well with surgical intervention and should not be
excluded on the basis of age. In orthopaedics the use of spinal anaethesia and
more efficient internal fixation, which can be inserted rapidly, have decreased
post-operative mortality. In all patients who fall, sustaining a fracture,
'sinister' causes must be excluded, including IHD, arrhythmia, CVA, sepsis
and increasing confusion.

Answer 6   **Marks**

(a)   Hypothermia
        Environmental – malnutrition, poor heating
        Hypothyroidism
        Sepsis
        CVA
        Drug overdose   3

(b)   FBC, U+Es, glucose, amylase, CK-MB, TFTs, blood cultures
        CXR
        ECG
        MSU
        ABGs   3

(c)   IV access
        Protect the airways
        IV fluids (cautiously)

IV antibiotics
Treat the underlying cause
Warm the patient slowly – blankets, warmed fluids
Subcutaneous heparin (unless contraindicated)   4

Comment

Hypothermia is defined as a core temperature below 35°C. Any patient presenting with an axillary or oral temperature below 35°C, should have a rectal temperature performed with a low reading thermometer. The elderly are particularly prone to hypothermic events due to environmental and systemic factors, and loss of thermoregulatory control mechanisms. It usually arises as a result of another major pathology, e.g. CVA, MI, falls or sepsis, although it may occur in isolation, particularly in the winter months. Whatever the cause, it generally has a poor prognosis in this age group, and carries a 50% mortality once core temperature falls to below 32°C. Treatment should be directed at the underlying cause, and the slow warming of the patient, the aim being to increase the core temperature at a rate of 0.5°C per hour. Intravenous fluids should be given cautiously, as they may precipitate pulmonary oedema; they should be warmed. Even when sepsis is not the principal cause of presentation, it is almost invariable in the unconscious, elderly patient, and it is recommended that they are given empirical broad spectrum antibiotics. The elderly are also at risk from thromboembolic disease and should be given prophylactic subcutaneous heparin.

Answer 7   **Marks**

(a)   Symptoms of the underlying disease, i.e. prostatism,
       retention, incontinence
       Gastrointestinal – nausea, vomiting, constipation, appetite,
       weight loss
       Pain – site, character, radiation, relieving and exacerbating
       factors
       Insomnia
       Mood   3

(b)   Anti-androgenics – cyproterone
       Analgesics – simple, combinations, opiates
       Steroids
       Antiemetics
       Night sedation
       Laxatives and enemas   3

(c)   Treatment of underlying disease – cyproterone, local
        radiotherapy, TURP
        Radiotherapy to bony metastases
        Palliation of specific symptoms, e.g. pain, depression, nausea,
        insomnia
        Specialist nurse and medical team involvement
        Family support
        Consider hospice care   4

Comment

Palliative care is an integral part of the treatment of the dying patient. With improvements in our understanding of the molecular and anatomical basis of disease, and the therapeutic options available, it has become a major speciality in its own right. The aims of therapy move away from curing the patient to alleviating distress, and allowing the terminal period, which may vary from days to months, to be as pleasant and dignified as possible. The major symptom categories which must be addressed, are:-

- **Gastrointestinal** – Appetite (may be improved by use of oral steroids); Nausea and vomiting; Constipation (commonly due to opiate analgesia, therefore usually foreseeable. Patients started on opiates should receive regular laxatives, and may require enemas and even manual evacuation); Dysphagia (may be due to the underlying disease, or candidiasis); Weight loss.
- **Pain** – as in any patient there is only one rule of analgesia and that is to 'be appropriate'. Until the patient is comfortable or pain free, one should consider all forms of analgesia. Simple – paracetamol, NSAIDs, Mechanical therapy – massage, reflexology, TENS; Combination – coproxamol, codydramol, aspav (aspirin and papaveretum); Opiates – MST, morphine elixir, subcutaneous infusion; Others – spinal and nerve blocks
- **Sleep** – sedation and appropriate analgesia usually allow the patient to sleep. However it must be remembered that some people are quite happy with 2–3 hours of sleep per night and should not be over-sedated for the staff's convenience!
- **Mood/psyche** – depression, denial, anger and exhaustion are all common symptoms, which are all exacerbated by poor palliation of the physical symptoms listed above.

Steroids often help with low mood and poor appetite, but antidepressants and psychiatric intervention may be needed.

SECTION III:
ESSAY WRITING

CHAPTER 1: STRUCTURED OUTLINES

QUESTION 1

A 69-year-old male smoker presents with a four-month history of a productive cough, episodic haemoptysis and exertional dyspnoea. Discuss the differential diagnosis, and your management of the most likely cause.

Plan

Differential diagnosis:

    bronchogenic carcinoma
    tuberculosis
    bronchiectasis
    multiple pulmonary emboli
    biventricular cardiac failure
    The most likely cause is a bronchogenic carcinoma

History: features of malignancy
Specific: hoarse voice (recurrent laryngeal nerve palsy)
     visual disturbance – Horner's syndrome
     paraesthesia and numbness along the ulnar border of the forearm and ulnar two fingers – brachial plexus invasion by Pancoast's tumour
     ectopic hormone secretion, e.g. SIADH and parathyroid hormone-like peptide
Non-specific: weight loss, anorexia, constipation, depression

Examination
General: clubbing of the finger nails, nicotine staining of the hands, cachexia, lymphadenopathy – supraclavicular, cervical and axillary
Respiratory examinations: signs of lobar collapse, consolidation and pleural effusions
Investigations: bloods – FBC, U+Es, LFTs, calcium and phosphate
     sputum – MC+S, AAFBs and cytology
     CXR
     bronchoscopy and biopsy
     +/– aspiration of pleural effusion and pleural biopsy
Therapeutic management is based on investigation results
Options: surgical excision +/– post-operative radiotherapy
     radiotherapy
     chemotherapy
     palliative care

QUESTION 2

What are the causes of cardiac failure? Discuss the management of a 54-year-old woman who presents with a six-month history of exertional dyspnoea, swollen ankles and three pillow orthopnoea.

Plan

Causes of cardiac failure:

acute – myocardial infarction causing left ventricular failure, mitral valve regurgitation and ventricular septal defect

arrythmia

bacterial endocarditis

pulmonary embolism

septicaemia and other causes of multiorgan failure

chronic – ischaemic heart disease

hypertension

idiopathic cardiomyopathy

valvular heart disease

cor pulmonale

Management: this woman's symptoms are suggestive of biventricular cardiac failure

History: specific symptoms of cardiac failure and causative disorders, e.g. angina

risk factors, e.g. hypertension, diabetes, peripheral vascular disease, smoking, alcohol, obesity and hyperlipidaemia

exacerbating factors – beta-blockers

Examination: signs of cardiac failure, e.g. tachycardia, gallop rhythm, raised jugular venous pressure, basal crepitations, peripheral oedema

Other signs: stigmata of hyperlipidaemia, cardiac murmurs, absent peripheral pulses

Investigations: bloods – FBC, U+Es, glucose, lipids, TFTs

CXR

ECG

echocardiogram

Therapeutic: general – treat underlying causes, remove exacerbating factors

address risk factors

specific – diuretics, ACE inhibitors

second line therapy, e.g. digoxin

surgical valve replacement or ventricular aneurysm resection

QUESTION 3

Write an essay on the causes and management of bloody diarrhoea in a 24-year-old woman.

Plan

Causes: infective – salmonella, shigella, amoebiasis, campylobacter, HIV related inflammatory bowel disease, ulcerative colitis and Crohn's disease
ischaemic colitis

Management:

History: duration of illness
diarrhoea – frequency, consistency, colour
blood – mixed or separate from stool, quantity
associated features – anorexia, weight loss, abdominal pain, nausea and vomiting
systemic features of IBD

Examination: general – clubbing, anaemia, jaundice, cachexia, pyrexia
abdominal masses, fistulae
PR examination – peri-anal disease

Investigation: FBC, U+Es, LFTs, ESR
AXR
stool specimen – MC+S, ova, parasites and cysts
sigmoidoscopy and biopsy

Therapeutic: based on the cause identified by investigation

QUESTION 4

Discuss the management of a 31-year-old woman who is found unconscious at home after taking an overdose of diazepam and paracetamol tablets.

Plan

Initial management: airway – protect and maintain the airway (will require anaesthetic help)
breathing
circulation – will need IV access and fluids started
cardiac monitor
pulse oxymetery
urinary catheter
cardiovascular, respiratory and neurological assessment

Initial investigations: FBC, U+Es, glucose, LFTs, clotting, drug levels – paracetamol and salicylates
CXR
ECG
ABGs

Therapeutic management: stomach washout, with protection of airway (this may not be applicable if prolonged period after overdose)
Diazepam: try flumazenil as a reversing agent for depression of consciousness
Paracetamol: toxic levels will indicate need for N-Acetyl – cysteine infusion
patient's hepatic and renal function must be closely followed with daily INR LFTs and U+Es
Once patient is medically well enough she will require psychiatric assessment

QUESTION 5

Write an essay on the causation and diagnosis of a first epileptic seizure in a 48-year-old woman. What therapeutic options could you use to treat her?

Plan

Causes: primary/idiopathic epilepsy – less likely in this age group
      secondary –   malignant brain tumour
                metastases – carcinoma of the lung or breast
                lymphoma
                intracerebral haemorrhage and thrombo-embolic stroke
                subdural haemorrhage
                intracerebral abscess

Clinical examination: signs of systemic disease
                papilloedema
                localizing neurological signs

Investigations: bloods – FBC and differential, clotting, ESR, blood cultures (if appropriate)
            CXR
            CT or MRI head scan
            EEG

Therapeutic options:
Idiopathic: anti-epileptics – first line: carbamazepine, sodium valproate
            second line treatment: phenytoin
            add on therapy – vigabatrin, lamotrigine, gabapentin
Secondary causes:
            tumours – neurosurgical excision + post-operative radiotherapy
                radiotherapy
                chemotherapy
            abscess – neurosurgical incision and drainage with post-operative IV antibiotics
            subdural haemorrhage – neurosurgical drainage
            thromboembolic stroke – anticoagulation

CHAPTER 2: MODEL ESSAYS

QUESTION:

Write an essay on the diagnosis and management of a 56-year-old man who presented to the Accident and Emergency Department having vomited two cupfuls (200 ml) of fresh blood a few hours previously.

ANSWER 1 – A COMFORTABLE PASS

Introduction
Chronic peptic ulceration (gastric and duodenal ulcers) accounts for approximately half of all cases of upper gastrointestinal haemorrhage. Other causes are bleeding from gastro-oesophageal varices (<5%), refux oesophagitis (5%), Mallory–Weiss syndrome (5–10%), acute gastric ulcers and erosions (20%) and, rarely, gastric carcinoma. Other uncommon causes are hereditary telangiectasia, pseudo xanthoma elasticum and blood dyscrasias. Aspirin and other non-steroidal anti-inflamatory agents along with alcohol intake produce bleeding from acute ulcers and these agents make chronic ulcers more likely to bleed.

Initial Management
The patient had suffered a recent significant though non-catastrophic upper gastrointestinal haemorrhage and must be admitted to hospital. He would be expected to pass the remaining blood as melaena over the ensuing days. A loss of up to a litre of blood in a previously healthy individual under the age of 60 years is readily compensated haemodynamically and no immediate resuscitatory measures are required. Bedrest and sedation (as anxiety compounds haemorrhage) with blood grouped and cross-matched with establishment of a venous access line and monitoring of vital signs are sufficient immediate measures. A detailed history and physical examination is carried out along with a peripheral blood profile.

Investigations
The diagnosis may be obvious from the history, e.g. a long history of dyspepsia or, more significantly, previous haemorrhage from a peptic ulcer. A history of aspirin or non-steroidal anti-inflammatory drug ingestion would suggest acute ulceration. Signs of chronic liver disease, viz. hepato-splenomegaly or stigmata of portal hypertension would suggest a variceal bleed, but occasionally it may occur from an accompanying peptic ulcer in patients with chronic liver disease.

An upper GI endoscopy (flexible oesophago-gastro-duodenoscopy) will detect the cause of the haemorrhage in over 80% of cases. If evidence of a recent bleed is seen, i.e. a visible vessel or an adherent clot, the patient is more likely to rebleed. A low haemoglobin level would suggest chronic blood loss prior to the haematemesis that brought the patient to hospital.

Treatment
Once the cause of the bleeding is identified, treatment measures may be instituted. If an acute bleeding source is visualized at endoscopy the bleeding may be arrested by submucosal injection of 1:200,000 solution of adrenaline or by electro-coagulation with a heater probe or by photo-coagulation with an ND-YAG (yttrium argon gun) laser. The patient is then placed on omeprazole or H_2 receptor blockade which promotes mucosal healing by inhibiting acid secretion. H_2 receptor antagonists – cimetidine or ranitidine are the first line of treatment of a chronic duodenal ulcer. A divided dose during the day with doubling of the dose at bedtime produces an over 80% reduction in acid secretion with an over 80% incidence of ulcer healing after a two-month course. Once ulcer healing is confirmed at endoscopy the patient may be advised either to continue treatment on a low-dose maintenance regime or to repeat the course if symptoms recur. Duodenal ulcers showing poor healing with H_2 receptor blockers may be treated with omeprazole, with ulcer healing rates of nearly 100% after four weeks' treatment. Sucralfate is occasionally used and works by protecting the mucosa by coating it against the acid. If evidence of *Helicobacter pylori* infection is detected, an H_2 receptor blocker is combined with metronidazole and amoxycillin or tetracycline for a six-week period.

H_2 receptor antagonists are also the first choice in the treatment of a chronic gastric ulcer, although they are less effective in promoting healing. Proton pump inhibitors are, therefore, increasingly used as initial therapy but if rebleeding occurs surgery is indicated if endoscopic measures fail. Peptic ulceration caused by gastrin producing tumours of the pancreas is severe and recurrent. Surgical resection of the tumour may not be curative if these are multiple or have metastasized. Acid secretion may be suppressed by high doses of proton pump inhibitors or H_2 receptor blockade. In those who are non-compliant or non-responsive to medical therapy, total gastrectomy may be required.

The diagnosis of a malignant gastric ulcer is by endoscopic visualization and biopsy or barium meal examination. Surgical resection offers the only hope of a cure.

A Mallory–Weiss mucosal tear at the gastro-oesophageal junction is produced by coughing or retching and bleeding usually stops spontaneously; rarely the tear may require suture. Variceal haemorrhage may be controlled by endoscopic sclerotherapy or banding of the feeding submucosal veins in the oesophagus. Continued bleeding necessitates an intravenous infusion of vasopressin or somatostatin to reduce the splanchnic blood flow, and balloon tamponade with a Sengstaken–Blakemore tube. The latter is left *in situ* for a period of approximately 12 hours followed by re-endoscopy to confirm cessation of bleeding. Sucralfate is given to prevent oesophageal ulceration following sclerotherapy. Variceal bleeding that is uncontrolled by these means necessitates oesophageal transection with ligation of the feeding vessels. Endoscopic surveillance is used to detect and treat recurrent varices with a maintenance dose of oral propranolol to lower the resting pulse rate by 25% which reduces the incidence of rebleeding when the liver disease is well compensated.

General Lifestyle Measures
Smoking and alcohol consumption along with drugs that provoke mucosal erosions must be avoided. Regular eating habits with adequate rest must be encouraged along with ways of modifying stresses associated with modern-day living.

Examiner's comments:
- The essay is eminently readable, knowledgeable and concise with appropriate sub-divisions.
- The introduction defines the problem and its causes.
- Diagnosis is based on the history, examination and investigations with emphasis being rightly placed on the first and the last.
- The question is very broad and therefore treatment can only be covered in outline. However, clear guidelines on each treatment modality is given.
- The importance of endoscopy for diagnosis and surveillance and its use in treatment for specific lesions is stated.
- The need for long-term drug therapy for chronic lesions and the importance of general lifestyle measures is mentioned.

ANSWER 2 – AN ANSWER SHOWING INSUFFICIENT KNOWLEDGE

The diagnosis of this man should involve the following stages: History, Examination, Investigation, Treatment.

The history starts by asking for the mainly formal details, i.e. name, age, address, GP, date of birth. Next ask for the patient's presenting complaint and record this in the patient's own words. The history of the presenting complaint should involve a review of the relevant system, i.e. the patient is vomiting blood, so it is necessary to ask about how much blood, the colour of the blood, how long this has been going on for and if he has ever had this before.

Record the patient's past medical history including any operations he has had in the past and illnesses, e.g. high blood pressure, diabetes, epilepsy, rheumatic fever, jaundice and TB. Ask about the drug history and any allergic responses. Next consider the social history in which smoking and alcohol are very important. A common cause of haematemesis is excess alcohol consumption producing a Mallory–Weiss tear. Ask about the patient's housing arrangements and as the patient will undoubtedly have to be admitted it is important to look into who would take care of the household. Next ask about the family history. Review of systems should encompass respiratory, cardiovascular, gastrointestinal, urogenital and musculo-skeletal systems.

Examination of the patient which follows takes the following sequence: observation, palpation, percussion and auscultation.

Firstly, check for jaundice, anaemia, clubbing, cyanosis, oedema and lymphadenopathy. A full physical examination involving all the systems should follow.

Investigations are the next stage and should include a full blood count, liver function tests, a chest X-ray and blood grouped and cross-matched. A treatment plan is then formulated. The possible causes of this patient's haematemesis could be ulcer, mitotic lesion, trauma or alcohol abuse.

Intravenous access should be established and pain relief given. If the patient is feverish it would be necessary to administer antibiotics for a probable infective cause. An exact (definitive) diagnosis may be established when the investigations are to hand.

Examiner's comments:

- Shows a poor understanding of the question and knowledge required to answer it.
- The urgent need to establish the diagnosis is not appreciated.
- Despite some idea of the possible causes of the bleeding, the candidate has little idea how to identify the bleeding source.
- A good deal of time is wasted on an irrelevent history and examination.
- There is no mention of treatment of any of the possible causes, nor follow-up.

ANSWER 3 – AN ANSWER SHOWING INSUFFICIENT KNOWLEDGE

The initial stage of the diagnostic procedure is a complete history expressly concentrating on previous episodes, bleeding tendencies, current medication, recent history of vomiting prior to haematemesis, ingestion of alcohol, symptoms of liver disease or peptic ulcer.

Examination would entail (i) pulse, blood pressure ventilation rate, (ii) signs of anaemia or chronic blood loss, (iii) stigmata of liver disease, (iv) guarding with signs of peritonitis and (v) a rectal examination to exclude rectal bleeding.

Investigations include a full blood count, urea and electrolytes, liver function tests and grouping, cross-matching and saving in case of continued bleeding. Most importantly an endoscopic examination of the oesophagus down to the duodenum to identify a bleeding lesion such as ruptured varices or a Mallory–Weiss tear at the gastro-oesophageal junction or a bleeding ulcer in the stomach or duodenum.

A bleeding vessel can be injected with a sclerosant, such as phenol, or sealed by diathermy or laser. If varices are involved a Sengstaken tube can be passed down and inflated to compress the bleeding source.

Admit and refer to the gastroenterologist; if the cause is traumatic a surgeon may be required.

An important omission is not to prepare for the possibility of shock should the bleeding recur, i.e. establish IV access and rehydrate with normal saline and/or colloids while blood is being cross-matched.

Examiner's comments:
*   Is aware of the urgent nature of the condition and has some idea of the possible causative lesions.
*   Shows some knowledge of the lesions involved but is insufficient in depth.
*   No mention of the treatment of the commonest lesion, viz peptic ulcer/erosions.
*   No mention of follow-up and the management of recurrence.

ANSWER 4 – AN ANSWER SHOWING INSUFFICIENT KNOWLEDGE

The initial management of a patient presenting with haematemesis is to assess his volaemic status. The volume of blood vomited will not be a good indicator of total blood loss, as estimates by the patient will be inaccurate as not all blood will be vomited.

Initial observations of blood pressure, pulse and respiratory rate should be made looking for signs of shock. If this is present the patient should be laid flat, intravenous access established and an infusion of a plasma expander such as gelofusin started. Even if shock is not present at presentation IV access should be established and blood grouped and saved in case of further bleeding. Observations of BP and pulse should be continued.

Once the patient is stable, a history should be taken. Pertinent questions on the presenting complaint include: time of haematemesis in relation to presentation, the volume and nature of blood in vomit; any associated symptoms; previous episodes and melaena or a history of alcohol abuse, smoking, liver failure or peptic ulcer.

On examination, as well as looking for signs of shock, look for stigmata of chronic liver disease. A PR examination should be performed for evidence of melaena.

Appropriate investigations are a full blood count; a low Hb would indicate chronic bleeding. Bleeding two hours previously is unlikely to produce a drop in Hb as a shift of fluid into the intravascular compartment will not yet have occurred. In addition a slightly raised MCV could indicate a reticulocytosis, further supporting chronic bleeding. A low platelet count could indicate thrombocytopaenia and a bleeding tendency. LFTs for evidence of liver failure; clotting screen for a bleeding tendency; also supports evidence of liver failure. A differential diagnosis would include bleeding oesophageal varices; Mallory–Weiss tear; severe reflux oesophagitis; eroded peptic ulcer; ulcerating gastric carcinoma and trauma.

In distinguishing between these possibilities evidence of liver failure would point towards varices. This is the diagnosis to be differentiated as it is an indication for urgent endoscopy. If this shows varices the bleeding may be controlled by injecting the varices.

If varices are thought to be unlikely the patient should be admitted to an acute bed and kept under observation for signs of shock or further blood loss. If this occurs transfusion should be considered, combined with plasma expanders if necessary. The patient should be kept nil by mouth. Endoscopy should be arranged as soon as possible to make the definitive diagnosis of the cause of bleeding. Many of the causes can now be corrected by endoscopy.

Examiner's comments:
- Too much preoccupation with shock which kept recurring through the essay.
- The urgent nature of the presentation is appreciated.
- The need for constant monitoring is appreciated.
- The commonest cause for the bleeding, viz peptic ulcer/erosion is not recognized.
- The treatment of variceal bleeding is inadequate.
- The treatment of all other causes are not mentioned.
- An inadequate knowledge of OGD as a diagnostic and therapeutic tool.

ANSWER 5 – AN ANSWER SHOWING INSUFFICIENT KNOWLEDGE

The patient should be brought into a cubicle and note should be taken of any obvious signs of anaemia or illness. A full history should be taken with particular emphasis on the amount of blood loss and its colour and if the patient experienced pain with the vomiting, viz Mallory–Weiss tear. Had the patient any chest or abdominal pain at other times and whether there was a history of trauma. A poor diet or the intake of spicy food and alcohol intake may predispose to ulcers, along with smoking. A drug history with particular emphasis on the use of pain-killers, viz anti-inflammatory drugs. Any previous episodes should be enquired.

Examination should then follow; first pulse, BP and respiratory rate are measured looking for shock. Then the abdominal system is of principal concern and the following points are of principal interest: the presence or absence of stigmata of chronic liver disease; the presence of anaemia; lymphadenopathy, viz Virchow's node (gastric Ca); any areas of abdominal tenderness; any abdominal masses viz. organomegaly (spleen, liver, kidneys); signs of portal hypertension; a per rectal examination should be undertaken.

Investigations should then follow; blood should be taken looking at full blood count and ESR (for possible anaemia and infection); U+Es, liver function tests and for grouping, saving and cross-matching. A chest X-ray to look for trauma, etc. Eventually the patient will be sent for endoscopy to try to locate the source of the bleeding, the patient being admitted for these investigations.

Once these investigations are underway therapeutic options may be taken depending on what is found. Bleeding varices usually require endoscopic intervention as an emergency; they can be injected or compressed. Ulcers that have perforated can be surgically resected.

Examiner's comments:
- A poorly planned attempt with disorganised thoughts.
- The urgent nature of the presentation is appreciated and the possible need for resuscitation.
- Endoscopy was the last in the sequence of investigations despite realization that this was essential for a diagnosis of the cause.
- There is some knowledge of causative lesions though management of these is at best vague.
- There is no mention of the management of peptic ulcer/erosion, the commonest cause of the bleeding.

SECTION IV:
ESSAY QUESTIONS

Essay Questions

INFECTIONS

1. Describe how you would investigate a male patient aged 22 with apparent candidiasis infection in the mouth, who had also recently lost weight and become breathless.

2. Discuss the epidemiology, clinical course and possible prevention of Hepatitis B infection.

3. Describe the clinical manifestations of infection with HIV.

   What methods are available for: (a) preventing the spread and (b) modifying the course of the disease?

4. What are primary, secondary and tertiary prevention? Giving as an example any communicable disease, describe the prevention strategies for each of the three categories.

5. Compare the causative organisms of bacterial meningitis in the neonate, child and adult. Discuss the management in a 9-year-old girl who is admitted with meningococcal meningitis.

6. What do you understand by the term 'septicaemic shock'? Discuss the common causes and the general principles of your management.

METABOLIC DISEASES

1. Malnutrition complicates many illnesses in an affluent society but is often unrecognized and untreated. Discuss possible reasons why this aspect of disease may be neglected and suggest possible steps that may be taken to prevent diseases associated with nutritional excess.

2. Define obesity. Discuss the relative values of the different methods used to assess the degree of obesity. Describe your regimen for the treatment of simple obesity in a woman of 35 years.

3. Discuss the investigation and management of a 43-year-old man with hypercholesterolaemia.

4. Discuss how you would counsel parents of a child with a newly diagnosed autosomal recessive metabolic disorder of your choice.

Discuss the prognosis, treatments and the diagnostic tests available.

5.   Compare and contrast haemochromatosis with Wilson's disease.

NEUROLOGY

1.   Describe the clinical features of migraine and the differential diagnosis from other types of headaches. How would you manage a patient with migraine?

2.   Discuss the clinical manifestations of multiple peripheral neuropathy and their relation to the aetiology.

3.   Discuss the causes of a facial nerve palsy, and the management of one cause.

4.   How would you manage a young woman newly diagnosed with generalized tonic-clonic seizure?

5.   A woman of 70 wakes one morning with weakness in her right arm and difficulty with speech. How would you arrive at a diagnosis and what are the probable causes? How would you counsel the patient and her relatives?

6.   Discuss how you would investigate and manage a 26-year-old man who presents with an episode of painful, blurred vision and numbness in his hands and feet.

ENDOCRINOLOGY

1.   Write an essay on the clinical manifestations and treatment of acromegaly.

2.   What conditions may present with the symptom of thirst? What investigations would you carry out on such a patient?

3.   Describe the clinical presentation of myxoedema. What investigations would you require to confirm the diagnosis, and how would you treat a 68-year-old woman with this condition?

4.   Write an essay on the pathogenesis of primary, secondary and tertiary

hypercalcaemia. What are the principles of treatment in each of these conditions?

5. Write an essay on the clinical manifestations of overactivity and under-activity of the adrenal cortex.

6. Discuss the management of mild, uncomplicated diabetes mellitus in the different age groups.

RESPIRATORY MEDICINE

1. Discuss the major differences in history, examination and investigations between the common and atypical pneumonias. Give a brief account of the complications of pneumococcal pneumonia.

2. Describe the management of an acute attack of asthma in a 25-year-old woman.

3. To what can the present rise in the incidence of TB in this country be attributed? What factors may result in this trend being reversed?

4. Write an essay on respiratory failure and its management.

5. Describe the diagnosis, management and clinical associations of pneumothorax.

CARDIOLOGY

1. Discuss the clinical features, diagnosis and management of a 16-year-old girl with infective endocarditis.

2. Write an essay on the complications and management of mitral stenosis.

3. Describe the clinical features of acute myocardial infarction and discuss the immediate management in a 58-year-old man.

4. Discuss the investigation and management of a 51-year-old man with essential hypertension.

5. Give an account of the clinical presentation, differential diagnosis and

treatment of acute pericarditis.

6. Describe the causes, clinical features and treatment of congestive cardiac failure.

HAEMATOLOGY

1. Discuss the diagnosis and treatment of iron deficiency anaemia. What factors may slow the response to treatment?

2. Give an account of the symptoms and signs to be found in a patient with pernicious anaemia. How would you treat this patient?

3. Write an essay on the hazards of blood transfusion. What are the features of a transfusion reaction and how would you manage such an event?

4. Give an account of the adult leukaemias. Discuss the investigations required to make a diagnosis and the common treatment modalities used.

5. Discuss the investigation and management of a patient with suspected multiple myeloma.

6. Discuss how you would investigate a patient with haemolytic anaemia; what are the features of chronic haemolytic disease?

DERMATOLOGY

1. What is the 'triple response' of the skin? In what conditions is it produced? How would you investigate and treat a case of urticaria?

2. Discuss the general principles of managing a patient with pruritus.

3. In what disorders and in what ways may hair growth be affected? How would you treat male-pattern baldness?

4. How would you manage a young adult presenting with psoriasis?

5. Write an essay on abnormalities of the nails.

Essay Questions

GASTROENTEROLOGY

1. A middle-aged man is brought into the Accident and Emergency department, having vomited a large quantity of blood, and feeling very weak and faint. Describe your immediate management and discuss the investigations required to arrive at a diagnosis.

2. Describe the factors underlying the formation of ascites. Discuss the principles of management when the ascites is due to chronic liver disease.

3. Discuss the investigation and management of a 45-year-old woman presenting with a two-month history of jaundice. (Ultrasound scan shows 'no gall stones present in the gall bladder'.)

4. Describe the clinical features and management of a 28-year-old woman suffering from acute ulcerative colitis.

5. Discuss the clinical presentation, investigations and management of a 24-year-old woman with coeliac disease, listing the differential diagnosis.

6. A 41-year-old man presents with symptoms suggestive of a duodenal ulcer. Discuss your investigation and management.

NEPHROLOGY

1. What are the clinical and biochemical features of 'end-stage' renal failure, and how may it be treated?

2. Discuss the aetiology and management of a young adult with acute glomerulonephritis.

3. Discuss the management of a 21-year-old woman who presents with recurrent urinary tract infections.

4. Discuss the genetics of polycystic kidney disease and outline its management and complications.

5. How would you assess a patient for renal transplantation and how would you prevent post-transplant rejection?

Essay Questions

RHEUMATOLOGY AND CONNECTIVE TISSUE DISEASES

1. Discuss the investigations and therapeutic management of a 29-year-old woman who presents with a bilaterally symmetrical polyarthropathy.

2. What impact has immunology made on the diagnosis of rheumatological and connective tissue diseases?

3. A 21-year-old woman presents with an acutely inflamed left knee. Discuss the likely causes and your management.

4. Compare and contrast the systemic vasculitides.

5. Discuss the clinical manifestations and management of a patient with systemic sclerosis.

PSYCHIATRY

1. What are the physical and mental features of severe anorexia nervosa? Discuss the treatment and prognosis.

2. What is a compulsive neurosis? Describe the features, predisposing factors and available treatment measures.

3. A wife reports that her 45-year-old husband is excessively jealous, accusing her of infidelity and threatening to harm her. How would you assess the situation, and advise both the husband and the wife?

4. What are the causes of acute mania and how may they be differentiated and treated?

5. 'Drug abuse is the scourge of the 20th Century'. How does it impinge on the community you live in? Discuss the measures you would adopt as a community physician to counteract this.

6. Write an essay on the social and psychological factors which may lead to attempted suicide in different age groups.

CARE OF THE ELDERLY

1. An 84-year-old woman presents with metastatic carcinoma of the breast. Discuss your investigation and management.

2. A 91-year-old independent man presents with recurrent falls. Discuss your investigations and management.

3. What do you understand by the term 'dementia'? How would you assess and manage a 70-year-old man who is complaining of forgetfulness?

4. An 81-year-old man is determined to go home to his 5th floor flat despite reservations by the hospital medical staff. Discuss how you would ensure that he manages successfully at home.

5. An 80-year-old woman is admitted with mild heart failure, which responds well to treatment. However, after 3 days in hospital she becomes increasingly confused. Describe how you would investigate and manage this development.

APPENDIX A: THE EXAMINATION IN MEDICINE

Assessment of clinical competence

Medical training encompasses a wide range of complex and varied activities and has evolved to match the diverse abilities required of the practising clinician. Maintaining these skills is essential for the establishment of professional standards of excellence and satisfying public expectation.

Assessment of clinical competence over such a broad field is fraught with difficulty: it has to examine the results of a number of years of study, covering a large syllabus in a uniform, efficient, competent and reliable fashion. It should ensure that candidates who have achieved the required level of proficiency pass, and those who have not should fail. The examination should be seen by students and examiners as being fair.

The perfect examination not only has to accurately assess knowledge and understanding but also evaluate the powers of analysis in problem solving and decision making. In the clinical field to these attributes must be added the candidate's attitude to patients and clinical work, as well as their personal and professional development and conduct.

Why examine?

Over the last few decades a number of groups have questioned the need for formal assessment and have proposed continued, faculty-based evaluation in medical education. Nevertheless, the vast majority of medical schools and universities rely on staged examinations, to ensure the acquisition of a minimal knowledge base. Satisfactory performance may be accompanied by graduation, certification, and the right to practise. The level of achievement may influence progress and promotion.

Examinations are also valuable for students and teachers to establish personal and departmental standards, and one of the problems of statutory examinations is usually their lack of feedback of the details of a candidate's performance. Internal faculty examinations can be an aid to learning and a means of self-evaluation: this will become of increasing importance with the extension of continued medical education, to help students identify a weakness of personal knowledge and of teaching material. Even the most ardent supporters of continuous assessment cannot deny the stimulus and motivation of an examination, and it does separate good from bad candidates.

What system?

To justify their existence examinations have to be seen to be fair and linked with both the training and its stated objectives. Traditional medical examinations have been based on the essay, the oral and the clinical. History and examination are central to a doctor-patient relationship, and the clinical has held its ground in undergraduate and postgraduate assessment, although the division between medicine, surgery and other disciplines has often become blurred, the emphasis being on the history and examination rather than the underlying disorder. Short cases in some schools have been replaced or supplemented by Objective Structured Clinical Examinations (OSCEs) to accompany the written part, and orals have been restricted to distinction and borderline candidates.

The essay has come under the greatest scrutiny. Students and examiners have questioned the effectiveness of an essay paper, since the limited number of topics and the possible choice have encouraged students to spot questions and concentrate on only part of the syllabus. The marking of essays is time-consuming and unreliable. There may be variation in an individual examiner's reassessment of papers, as well as between examiners. The variation makes comparison at a national level difficult, and this is further accentuated by what has been described as the deep psychological reluctance of examiners to allocate more than 70% of the total marks allowed for any given essay question.

Attempts to modify the essay included modified essay questions (MEQs), which introduce a larger number of questions with a patient vignette, and a variety of sub-sections based on various aspects of diagnosis and treatment. Multiple short answers on a range of topics have also gained favour in some schools. Structured answer questions (SAQs) are a further development of the written assessment, testing problem solving and decision making in a struc-tured and objective fashion. They are proving a reliable means of assessing knowledge and understanding in clinical practice.

MCQs also have a wide application in medical assessment, having the potential of covering a wide body of knowledge and, in their extended matching pairs format, introducing reasoned responses rather than item recall. A computerised marking system has eased the examiners' burden in this section. A current trend in the written part of the clinical examination is to include both MCQs and SAQs, the former to determine the candidate's knowledge, and the latter to assess the application of this knowledge by reasoning, interpretation, problem-solving and decision-making.

SAQs
SAQs test the candidate's high-level skills rather than factual recall. They consist of a clinical vignette followed by two to four questions, which may

have sub-sections, with an indication of the marks allocated for each correct answer. The choice of scenario is based on common clinical problems pertinent and relevant to the field of study, and covering important concepts and principles relating to the course material. There is no room for trivia, irrelevant or esoteric topics, or interesting rarities.

Clinical information is presented in an ordered fashion, usually describing the history and examination, with or without investigations, of a specific condition. Questions should be clear, unambiguous and requiring the examinee to analyse and make decisions based on the given information. This may involve diagnosis or treatment and may also cover aspects of psychological, social and family history, and ethical issues.

Examiners are given a model answer and a marking schedule that has to be closely adhered to. Marking is time-consuming: allotting a single examiner to each question streamlines the process and allows uniformity of marking for a group of candidates. Any allowances made for near-misses will also be generalised. It is common to double mark a number of scripts to check examiners' inter-rater reliability across the whole examination.

Examiners preparing SAQs should form a panel, draw up a list of topics and allocate these topics among the group. The first draft of each question is read out at a group meeting, and comments made on the content, style, the importance, relevance and its educational standard.

The second draft of the questions is tried on a group of students under examination conditions, noting the time taken to complete four to eight questions. The answers are analysed and questions again modified if there are obvious misunderstandings, or unexpected ease or difficulty. Misinterpretation of the stem may lead to an erroneous diagnosis. As the rest of the question is usually based on the stem, a candidate may go off at a tangent in all subsequent answers. The examiners must then make an informed decision in allocating marks for such mishaps, provided the conclusions reached are logical and not far removed from the expected answers. However, in inadequately vetted questions more than one diagnosis may be arrived at from the stem. In such circumstances the onus is firmly on the examiner to accommodate such unanticipated correct responses and mark them fairly.

The completed questions are retained in a question bank. They should be added to each year, attention being given to the choice, number and range of topics. These should match the weighting given to each part of the syllabus.

It may take three to five years to build up an adequate bank, after this time any break in security is of less importance.

The stem of a question can often be modified by changing the disease and superficial data, such as the sex, age and the timing of the symptoms. This process eases the generation of further questions and allows some degree of comparison of standards when they are being analysed. Questions should be under continuous reappraisal after each use, to assess their performance and discriminatory value. Marks can be influenced by poor quality of questions, poor knowledge of answers and errors within the marking system.

Each examination requires 10–12 questions to allow a broad assessment and to produce discriminatory differences between good and bad candidates. Each question used should be independent of the others. In qualifying examinations one expects a high pass rate, and a significant number of candidates may achieve distinction level. If this is an entry point to a distinction viva it may be more practical to limit the viva to those within one or two standard errors of the maximum mark obtained.

Essays

MCQs are used routinely in most qualifying and postgraduate examinations. Nevertheless, medicine is not as black and white as MCQs would suggest, and many brighter students are averse to this form of assessment. Similarly, although SAQs allow much wider coverage of the syllabus and more objectivity in the marking systems they also restrict the examiner to black or white rigid marking schemes. The limitations of these features are well known to every clinician who has gone over recent examinations with groups of students.

The essay does test a candidate's ability to collect and quantify material, and assesses their powers of original thought and creativity. It determines the candidate's ability to write clear and legible English, and some schools have felt that these qualities should be retained in their assessment. In spite of the expensive manpower required in marking essay questions, an essay does assess a candidate's depth of knowledge in a specified area and, in preparing for an essay paper, candidates have to acquire detailed knowledge of much of the syllabus.

Revision for the essay paper is linked with revision of the whole course. If a candidate's knowledge base is poor, he or she will rightly fail; but if it is sound, it is essential that their examination technique is good enough to ensure success. The ease of revision is based on previous knowledge and a good filing system which, if disease-based, provides a check list for each condition so that current knowledge can be written and then checked against books and stored material to identify deficiencies.

The candidate is expected to have read around topics and patient problems encountered during the clinical course, gaining information from lectures, reviews, and current papers, as well as text books. This information should be filed in an easily retrievable form, such as notes in the margins of text books, a card system, plenty of lists and clearly written pieces of paper. People vary in the amount of information they can remember at any one time. Any deficiency, however, can be easily reversed during revision, provided previous information was well organised and fully understood at the time it was collected.

Examiners at an undergraduate level are keen to pass candidates, to ensure that they can continue with their careers. However, medical examiners have an obligation to ensure that ignorant and potentially dangerous individuals are not let loose on a patient population. At a postgraduate level examiners have to ensure that a candidate has a comprehensive and in-depth knowledge of their subject: gaps are likely to be penalised.

Regardless of the level of the examination, essays on clinical subjects have a similar format. This is based on a disease or a clinical problem and includes questions on the aetiology, pathology, diagnosis, differential diagnoses, complications, assessment, management and treatment. Each question must be read fully and every word noted as they will have been constructed very carefully.

Although the words 'discuss' and a few synonyms imply a certain vagueness, the response must be precise and directed. Having read the question, the answer plan is based on the clinical data required. These will usually correspond to the check list used to revise each disease.

Diagnosis and differential diagnosis are based on only three sources of information: namely, the **history**, **examination** and **investigation**. If the diagnosis is given, it may require confirmation from the same three sources. Assessment means diagnosis (history, examination, investigation) but adds the dimension of **severity** of the problems encountered. Management is assessment plus treatment. Although the term may be loosely used, implying just treatment in some questions, it is worth writing a few sentences on confirmation of diagnosis and severity of the problem being treated. Treatment should not be restricted to medicine, as many other problems may require to be sorted out first. Other disciplines that may be involved, must be considered such as nursing, physiotherapy, occupational therapy, and drugs, chemotherapeutic agents and radiotherapy. Radiological intervention forms a major part of treatment in many diseases.

The plan outlining the areas to be covered can be in the answer book or on scrap paper. The plan should take three to six minutes for most essays and allows concentrated thought around the topic. On completion a line is drawn through it to imply to the examiner that there is more to come, and then construct the first few sentences of the introduction. This should imply an understanding of the topic, giving the examiner confidence that the essay is on the right track and, hopefully, is of a good standard.

There is much debate as to whether headings should be underlined and key words highlighted. This debate is more of a problem to the candidate than the examiner, who is more concerned as to whether the script is legible, and demonstrates knowledge and understanding of the question. Illegibility is an inherent problem with some individuals. Examiners go to considerable effort to give candidates the benefit of the doubt but illegibility can never camouflage ignorance, and candidates would be well advised to write at a rate at which the end product is guaranteed readable to the examiner.

Literacy and mastery of prose are more debatable. As much as examiners would wish medical graduates to be able to write skilfully and coherently, marks are predominantly awarded for factual knowledge and understanding of an essay topic. Success is, therefore, based on an appropriate plan and the development of each heading within it.

Medical schools and colleges rarely set regular essays during their courses, even when they use this means of final assessment. It is, therefore, appropriate for students who know they will be examined in this way to undertake preliminary practice. A series of essay questions has, therefore, been added after the SAQs section in each chapter.

There is a section on planning structural outlines as a preliminary to writing essays, and examples of good and poor answers with examiner's comments. These guidelines may be used in planning and writing essays. The relevant practical information will usually be found in the sectional answers and teaching aids, and essays may be swapped with a working partner or discussion group to act as examiners. Subsequently the plan, development, depth of knowledge, literary style and legibility is discussed. As the exams draw near, the pass standard becomes apparent, and essays can be accurately assessed by peer review.

Whatever examination system is chosen, it must be reliable, valid and discriminatory, and it should not be influenced by the subjective judgement of an examiner. The examination should be about the contents of a paper and not expertise or prior coaching in the chosen system. Nevertheless, it is essential to have prior exposure to the local examination system and be well versed in its technique. This text is intended to provide that exposure and to educate candidates in the techniques of SAQ and essay writing in the hope of easing their passage to qualification.

APPENDIX B:
SELF-ASSESSMENT SAQ PAPERS

The Structured Answer Questions in this book are arranged by subject, enabling the reader to focus on individual subject areas and to systematically address any weak areas of knowledge.

However, during revision it is also very valuable to sit authentic test papers. This will help you to become accustomed to working under strictly timed conditions and should also contribute towards making the exam itself a less stressful experience.

The authors have created twelve complete SAQ practice papers, each containing a representative range of topics.

Instructions

- There are 12 questions in each paper, to be answered in two hours.
- You should spend no more than 10 minutes on each question.
- The questions have been designed to promote succinct answers.
- Marks available for each section are indicated next to the questions.
- If you are asked for two answers and you give more than two the best two will be marked.

Paper 1   1.1, 4.1, 6.1, 9.1, 3.1, 2.3, 8.1, 10.1, 5.4, 12.9, 11.11, 3.16

Paper 2   4.2, 1.2, 6.2, 5.11, 9.2, 7.8, 11.5, 8.2, 10.2, 12.8, 11.10, 3.2

Paper 3   6.3, 4.3, 1.3, 5.10, 9.3, 7.7, 2.4, 12.7, 8.3, 10.3, 11.9, 3.3

Paper 4   9.4, 4.4, 5.9, 1.4, 6.4, 7.6, 10.2, 12.6, 13.2, 8.4, 11.8, 3.4

Paper 5   9.5, 4.5, 6.5, 5.8, 1.5, 7.5, 10.4, 12.5, 13.6, 11.7, 8.5, 3.5

Paper 6   13.1, 4.6, 6.6, 5.7, 9.6, 1.6, 7.4, 12.4, 11.7, 11.6, 10.4, 3.6

Paper 7   4.7, 13.2, 6.7, 5.6, 9.7, 7.4, 1.7, 2.6, 3.15, 11.5, 10.5, 3.7

Paper 8   6.8, 4.8, 13.3, 5.5, 9.8, 2.5, 3.14, 1.8, 11.4, 10.6, 8.6, 3.8

Paper 9   9.9, 4.9, 5.4, 13.4, 2.4, 7.3, 3.3, 11.3, 1.9, 8.7, 10.7, 3.9

Paper 10   5.3, 9.10, 2.3, 6.9, 13.5, 7.2, 9.10, 12.3, 8.8, 1.10, 10.8, 3.10

Paper 11   4.11, 2.2, 5.2, 6.10, 9.11, 13.6, 9.14, 12.2, 11.2, 10.9, 1.11, 3.11

Paper 12   2.1, 4.12, 5.1, 6.11, 7.1, 9.12, 13.7, 12.1, 9.13, 11.1, 3.12, 1.12

APPENDIX C: SELF-ASSESSMENT ESSAY QUESTION PAPERS

The essay questions in this book are arranged by subject, enabling the reader to focus on individual subject areas and to systematically address any weak areas of knowledge.

However, during revision it is also very valuable to sit authentic test papers. This will help you to become accustomed to working under strictly timed conditions and should also contribute towards making the exam itself a less stressful experience.

The authors have created twelve complete essay papers, each covering a representative range of topics.

Instructions

* There are 4 questions in each paper, to be answered in 2 hours 20 minutes.
* You should spend no more than 35 minutes on each question, and you are advised to spend the first five minutes formulating an outline for your answer.

Paper 1   1.3, 4.3, 6.3, 9.3

Paper 2   2.3, 3.4, 5.2, 10.5

Paper 3   1.1, 7.2, 8.3, 2.1

Paper 4   3.2, 4.1, 6.1, 11.1

Paper 5   2.6, 5.1, 6.6, 8.1

Paper 6   1.5, 6.2, 4.5, 9.2

Paper 7   2.2, 5.4, 9.4, 10.1

Paper 8   1.4, 6.3, 4.4, 13.1

Paper 9   3.4, 5.5, 9.5, 10.2

Paper 10   1.6, 6.4, 4.6, 13.3

Paper 11   6.5, 3.6, 4.2, 9.6

Paper 12   1.2, 3.1, 5.3, 9.1

PASTEST BOOKS FOR UNDERGRADUATES

PasTest are the specialists in study guides and revision courses for professional medical qualifications. For over 30 years we have been helping doctors to achieve their potential. The PasTest range of books for medical students includes:

Essential MCQs for Medical Finals , Second edition
Rema Wasan, Delilah Hassanally, Balvinder Wasan   ISBN 1 901198 20 0

Essential MCQs for Surgical Finals, Second edition
Delilah Hassanally, Rema Singh   ISBN 1 901198 15 4

Essential MCQs in Clinical Pharmacology
Delilah Hassanally, Rema Singh   ISBN 1 901198 32 4

Essential MCQs in Obstetrics and Gynaecology
Dianah Hamilton-Fairley   ISBN 1 901198 34 0

EMQs for Medical Students Volume 1
A Feather et al   ISBN 1 901198 65 0

EMQs for Medical Students Volume 2
A Feather et al   ISBN 1 901198 69 3

OSCEs for Medical Undergraduates Volume 1
Adam Feather, Ramanathan Visvanathan, John SP Lumley   ISBN 1 901198 04 9

OSCEs for Medical Undergraduates: Volume 2
Adam Feather, Ramanathan Visvanathan, John SP Lumley   ISBN 1 901198 05 7

Medical Finals: Passing the Clinical
Christopher Moore, Anne Richardson   ISBN 1 901198 43 6

Surgical Finals: Passing the Clinical, Second edition
John SP Lumley,Gina Kuperberg   ISBN 1 901198 77 4

Surgical Finals: Structured Answers and Essay Questions
Ramanathan Visvanathan, John SP Lumley   ISBN 1 901198 43 X

Learning by Lists for Medical Students
Stuart McPherson   ISBN 1 901198 30 8

PasTest Books for Undergraduates

**The Practical Guide to Medical Ethics and Law for Junior Doctors
and Medical Students**
Chloe-Maryse Baxter, Mark Brennan, Yvette Coldicott   ISBN 1 901198 76 6

Radiology Casebook for Medical Students
Rema Wasan, Alan Grundy, Richard Beese   ISBN 1 901198 40 5

Clinical Skills for Medical Students: A Hands-on Guide
Ian Bickle, David McCluskey, Barry Kelly   ISBN 1 901198 86 3

How to order:
www.pastest.co.uk
To order books safely and securely online, shop at our website

Telephone: +44 (0)1565 752000
For priority mail order and have your credit card to hand when you call

Delivery to your door
With a busy lifestyle, nobody enjoys walking to the shops for something that may
or may not be in stock. Let us take the hassle and deliver direct to your door. We
will dispatch your book within 24 hours of receiving your order